Cardiovascular Care

made
Incredibly
Visual!®

Third Edition

Cardiovascular Care

made Incredibly Visual!

Third Edition

Clinical Editor

Mary Ann Siciliano McLaughlin, Ed.D., RN
Assistant Professor and Program Director
Accelerated BSN Program (Philadelphia campus)
Gwynedd Mercy University
Gwynedd Valley, Pennsylvania

. Wolters Kluwer

Philadelphia • Baltimore • New York • London
Buenos Aires • Hong Kong • Sydney • Tokyo

Acquisitions Editor: Nicole Dernoski
Developmental Editor: Maria M. McAvey
Editorial Coordinator: Lindsay Ries
Production Project Manager: Kim Cox
Design Coordinator: Elaine Kasmer
Manufacturing Coordinator: Kathleen Brown
Marketing Manager: Linda Wetmore
Prepress Vendor: SPi Global

3rd edition

Printed in China

Library of Congress Cataloging-in-Publication Data
Names: McLaughlin, Mary Ann Siciliano, 1968- editor.
Title: Cardiovascular care made incredibly visual! / clinical editor Mary Ann Siciliano McLaughlin.
Description: 3rd edition. | Philadelphia : Wolters Kluwer, [2018] | Includes bibliographical references and index.
Identifiers: LCCN 2017051525 | ISBN 9781496363374
Subjects: | MESH: Cardiovascular Diseases—nursing | Diagnostic Techniques, Cardiovascular—nursing | Handbooks | Atlases
Classification: LCC RC674 | NLM WY 49 | DDC 616.1/2025—dc23 LC record available at https://lccn.loc.gov/2017051525

RRS1711

Dedication

"People who love what they do wear themselves down doing it, they even forget to wash or eat."

Marcus Aurelius, Meditations, p. 53

I would like to dedicate this book to my three children—Erica, Elena, and JJ McLaughlin. I hope you love what you do each day in your future professions. I truly love being a nurse and teaching nursing. My hope is that you all find a passion similar to mine for nursing in your lifetime.

All my love,
Mom

Contributors

Diane M. Allen, PhD, ANP, BC, CLS
Adult Nurse Practitioner
Womack Army Medical Center
Fort Bragg, North Carolina

Madelyn Danner, RN, MSN, CCRN, CEN
Associate Professor of Nursing
Harford Community College
Bel Air, Maryland

Angela Kelly, DNP, RN, APN, WHNP-BC, RNC-OB
Clinical Assistant Professor
Rutgers School of Nursing–Camden
Camden, New Jersey

Jaime Mendiola, RN, MSN, CCRN, ACNP
Professor of Nursing
Bakersfield College
Bakersfield, California

Shafeah Morrison, DNP, ARNP, APN-C, FNP-BC
Family Nurse Practitioner, Optum Health
Faculty, Simmons College of Nursing, On-
 line; South University
Pembroke Pines, Florida

Lynn M. Simko, PhD, RN, CCRN
Clinical Associate Professor
School of Nursing
Duquesne University
Pittsburgh, Pennsylvania

Previous Edition Contributors

Diane M. Allen, RN, MSN, ANP, BC, CLS

Ellen Cummings, MSN, RN, CNRN

Madelyn Danner, RN, MSN, CCRN, CEN

Sophia Dixon, BSN, MS, CVN

Nancy Emma, RN, MSN

Margaret J. Malone, RN, MN, CCRN

Jaime Mendiola, RN, MSN, CCRN, ACNP

Lynn M. Simko, PhD, RN, CCRN

Dawn Zwick, RN, MSN, CRNP

Contents

Chapter 1

Anatomy and physiology

Location of the heart

The heart lies between the lungs and beneath the sternum within the mediastinum, or thoracic cage. The mediastinum is the "middle" section of the chest cavity that contains the tissues and organs and separates the two pleural sacs. In most people, two thirds of the heart extends to the left of the body's midline, close to the left midclavicular line. Inside the body, the heart is rotated so that its broad part, the base, is at its upper right and the pointed end, the apex, is at its lower left. The apex is the point of maximal impulse (PMI), where heart sounds are loudest.

Structures of the heart

Heart wall layers

- The *epicardium* (edge), the outer layer, is made up of squamous epithelial cells overlying connective tissue and serves as a protective layer.
- The *myocardium* (middle), the middle layer, is made up of striated muscle fibers and forms most of the heart wall. This muscle layer causes the heart to contract.
- The *endocardium* (inside), the inner layer, consists of endothelial tissue with small blood vessels and bundles of smooth muscle.

Anterior view

Pericardium
Fibrous pericardium
Serous pericardium
(parietal layer)

Serous pericardium
(visceral layer [epicardium])

Myocardium (muscle layer)

Endocardium

Superior vena cava
Pericardium
Left pulmonary artery
Aorta
Pulmonary trunk
Right atrium
Right ventricle
Left ventricle
Apex

A sac called the *pericardium* surrounds the heart and roots of the great vessels. It consists of two layers: the fibrous pericardium (tough, white fibrous tissue) and the serous pericardium (thin, smooth inner portion). The serous pericardium also has two layers: the parietal layer (lines the inside of the fibrous pericardium) and the visceral layer (adheres to the surface of the heart).

Between the fibrous and serous pericardium is the pericardial space. This space contains pericardial fluid, which lubricates the surfaces of the space and allows the heart to move easily during contraction.

Posterior view

Superior vena cava
Aortic arch
Left pulmonary artery
Right pulmonary artery
Right pulmonary veins
Left pulmonary veins
Left atrium
Right atrium
Inferior vena cava

Right ventricle
Left ventricle

Heart chambers

Within the heart lie four hollow chambers, two atria and two ventricles:
- The right and left atria serve as volume reservoirs for blood being sent into the ventricles.
- The interatrial septum divides the atrial chambers, helping them to contract and force blood into the ventricles below.
- The ventricles serve as the pumping chambers of the heart.
- The interventricular septum separates the ventricles and also helps them to pump.

Pump it up!

The thickness of a chamber's wall depends on the amount of high-pressure work the chamber does:
- Because the atria only have to pump blood into the ventricles, their walls are relatively thin.
- The walls of the **right ventricle** are thicker because it pumps blood against the resistance of the pulmonary circulation.
- The walls of the **left ventricle** are thickest of all because it pumps blood against the resistance of the systemic circulation.

Inside a normal heart

Superior vena cava

Branches of right pulmonary artery

Right atrium

Right pulmonary veins

Tricuspid valve

Chordae tendineae

Interventricular septum

Right ventricle

Papillary muscle

Inferior vena cava

Descending aorta

Aortic arch

Pulmonic valve

Branches of left pulmonary artery

Left atrium

Left pulmonary veins

Mitral valve

Aortic valve

Left ventricle

The more a muscle works, the larger it becomes.

Heart valves

The heart contains four valves: two atrioventricular (AV) valves (the mitral and tricuspid) and two semilunar valves (the pulmonic and aortic). The valves are unidirectional and allow forward flow of blood through the heart and prevent backward flow. Blood flow in the heart is meant to only go one way. Heart valves will open and close in response to pressure gradients contained within the chamber. Once the pressure gradient is increased, the valve will open to allow for passage of the moving blood and will close once the pressure gradient is decreased. The tricuspid valve, or right AV valve, prevents backflow from the right ventricle into the right atrium. The mitral valve, also known as the *bicuspid* or *left AV valve*, prevents backflow from the left ventricle into the left atrium. The pulmonic valve, one of the two semilunar valves, prevents backflow from the pulmonary artery into the right ventricle. The other semilunar valve is the aortic valve, which prevents backflow from the aorta into the left ventricle.

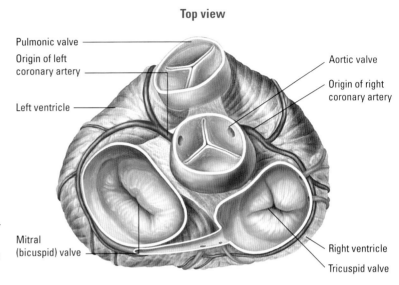

Top view

Pulmonic valve
Origin of left coronary artery
Left ventricle
Mitral (bicuspid) valve
Aortic valve
Origin of right coronary artery
Right ventricle
Tricuspid valve

The valves open to allow forward flow of blood through the heart. They immediately snap closed to prevent backward flow.

SNAP

Under pressure!

Pressure changes within the heart affect the opening and closing of the valves. The amount of blood stretching the chamber and the degree of contraction of the chamber wall determine the pressure. For example, as blood fills a chamber, the pressure rises; then, as the chamber wall contracts, the pressure rises further. This increase in pressure causes the valve to open and blood to flow out into an area of lower pressure, leading to an equal pressure state.

Flow of blood through the heart

Just like dancing a waltz, blood follows specific steps as it flows through the heart.

Step 1

Blood fills all heart chambers.
The right atrium receives deoxygenated blood returning from the body through the inferior and superior venae cava and from the heart through the coronary sinus. The left atrium receives oxygenated blood from the lungs through the four pulmonary veins. Passive filling of the ventricles begins with diastole.

Step 2

The atria contract. The remaining blood enters the ventricles.
The atria pump their blood through the two AV valves (mitral and tricuspid) directly into their respective ventricles.

memory board

BBRRLLL

Use this mnemonic to help you remember the flow of blood:

Barren **B**lood

Returns on the **R**ight

Loaded blood

Leaves on the **L**eft

Step 3

The ventricles contract. Blood enters the aorta and pulmonary arteries.
The right ventricle pumps blood through the pulmonic valve into the pulmonary arteries and then into the lungs. That blood returns, oxygenated, to the left atrium, completing pulmonic circulation.

The left ventricle pumps blood through the aortic valve into the aorta and then throughout the body. Deoxygenated blood returns to the right atrium, completing systemic circulation.

Cardiac conduction

The conduction system of the heart begins with the heart's pacemaker: the sinoatrial (SA) node. When an impulse leaves the **SA node**, it travels through the atria along Bachmann's bundle (the interatrial tract) and the internodal pathways on its way to the AV node. After the impulse passes through the AV node, it travels to the ventricles, first down the bundle of His, then along the bundle branches, and, finally, down the Purkinje fibers.

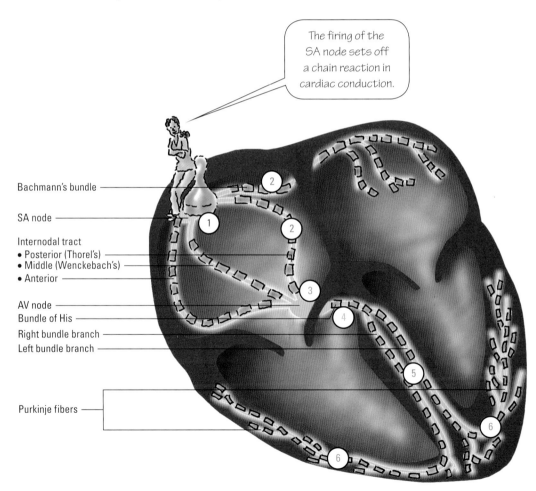

The firing of the SA node sets off a chain reaction in cardiac conduction.

Bachmann's bundle

SA node

Internodal tract
• Posterior (Thorel's)
• Middle (Wenckebach's)
• Anterior

AV node
Bundle of His
Right bundle branch
Left bundle branch

Purkinje fibers

Pacemakers of the heart

The SA node is the heart's primary pacemaker. Pacemaker cells in lower areas, such as the junctional tissue and the Purkinje fibers, initiate an impulse only when they don't receive one from above, such as when the SA node is damaged from a myocardial infarction.

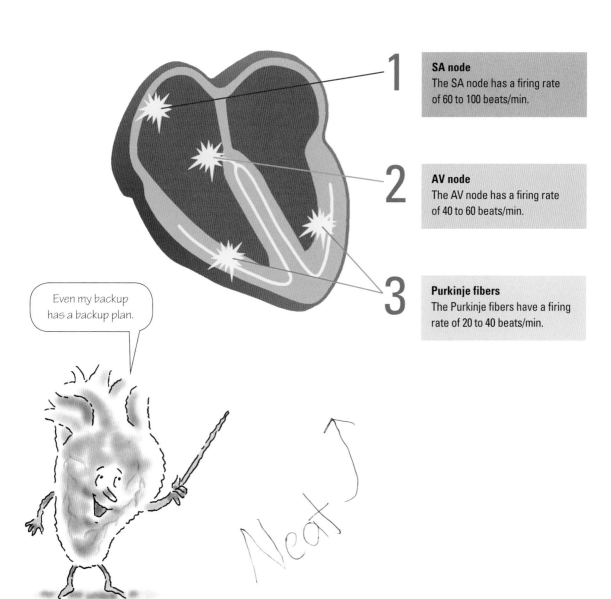

1 **SA node**
The SA node has a firing rate of 60 to 100 beats/min.

2 **AV node**
The AV node has a firing rate of 40 to 60 beats/min.

3 **Purkinje fibers**
The Purkinje fibers have a firing rate of 20 to 40 beats/min.

Generation and transmission of electrical impulses depend on four characteristics of cardiac cells.

Ability to spontaneously initiate an impulse (pacemaker cells have this ability)

A cell's response to an electrical stimulus (results from ion shifts across the cell membrane)

Ability of a cell to transmit an electrical impulse to another cardiac cell

Ability of a cell to contract after receiving a stimulus

Conduction junction

As impulses are transmitted, cardiac cells undergo cycles of depolarization and repolarization as described below.

Our hero, the heart, is at rest, with no electrical activity taking place. He's enjoying the state of being polarized.

But while he rests, negative charges flow in, disturbing his rest. While he's still resting, he has the potential to react. This is his resting potential.

Depolarization-repolarization cycle

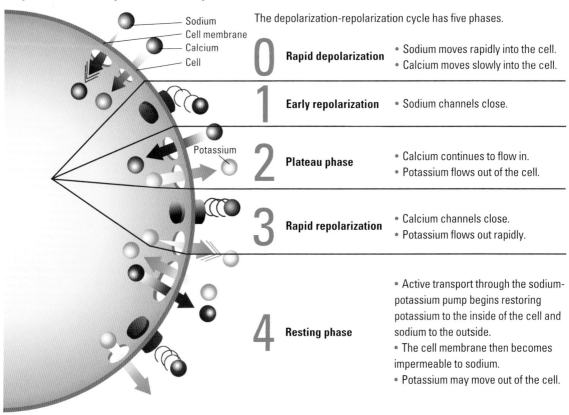

The depolarization-repolarization cycle has five phases.

0 **Rapid depolarization**
- Sodium moves rapidly into the cell.
- Calcium moves slowly into the cell.

1 **Early repolarization**
- Sodium channels close.

2 **Plateau phase**
- Calcium continues to flow in.
- Potassium flows out of the cell.

3 **Rapid repolarization**
- Calcium channels close.
- Potassium flows out rapidly.

4 **Resting phase**
- Active transport through the sodium-potassium pump begins restoring potassium to the inside of the cell and sodium to the outside.
- The cell membrane then becomes impermeable to sodium.
- Potassium may move out of the cell.

Diagram labels: Sodium, Cell membrane, Calcium, Cell, Potassium

Disturbed by a ringing SA node, the ions of his dreams start to flow into his muscles. He has the potential for action and jumps from the sofa. This is his action potential. His cells have depolarized.

Wrong number. Our hero attempts to return to his resting state by balancing his negative experience with positive thoughts. He's trying to repolarize.

Cardiac output

Cardiac output refers to the amount of blood the heart pumps in 1 minute. To determine cardiac output, multiply the heart rate by the stroke volume (the amount of blood ejected with each heartbeat). Stroke volume depends on three factors:

- preload
- contractility
- afterload.

Preload is the stretching of muscle fibers in the ventricles as the ventricles fill with blood. Think of preload as a balloon stretching as air is blown into it (the force of this stretch is preload). The more air being blown, the greater the stretch.

Contractility refers to the inherent ability of the myocardium to contract normally. Contractility is influenced by preload. The greater the stretch, the more forceful the contraction — or, the more air in the balloon, the greater the stretch, and the farther the balloon will fly when the air is allowed to expel.

Afterload refers to the pressure that the ventricular muscles must generate to overcome the higher pressure in the aorta to get the blood out of the heart. Resistance is the knot on the end of the balloon, which the balloon has to work against to get the air out.

Wonder how cardiac muscle contracts? Electrical stimulation causes troponin to expose actin-binding sites, which allows muscle contraction to occur.

Pulling it together

When a muscle cell is in the resting state, tropomyosin and troponin (a cardiac-specific protein) inhibit contractility by preventing actin-myosin binding.

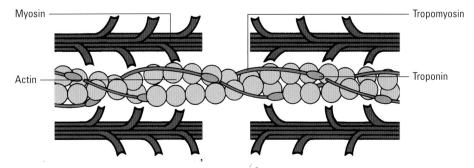

Electrical stimulation causes calcium release. Calcium binds to troponin, changing the configuration of tropomyosin and exposing actin-binding sites. Myosin and actin bind, creating cross-bridges, and the muscle contracts.

Cycle of heart sounds

When you auscultate a patient's chest and hear that familiar "lub-dub," you're hearing the first and second heart sounds: S_1 and S_2. At times, two other sounds may occur: S_3 and S_4.

Heart sounds are generated by events in the cardiac cycle. When valves close or blood fills the ventricles, vibrations of the heart muscle can be heard through the chest wall.

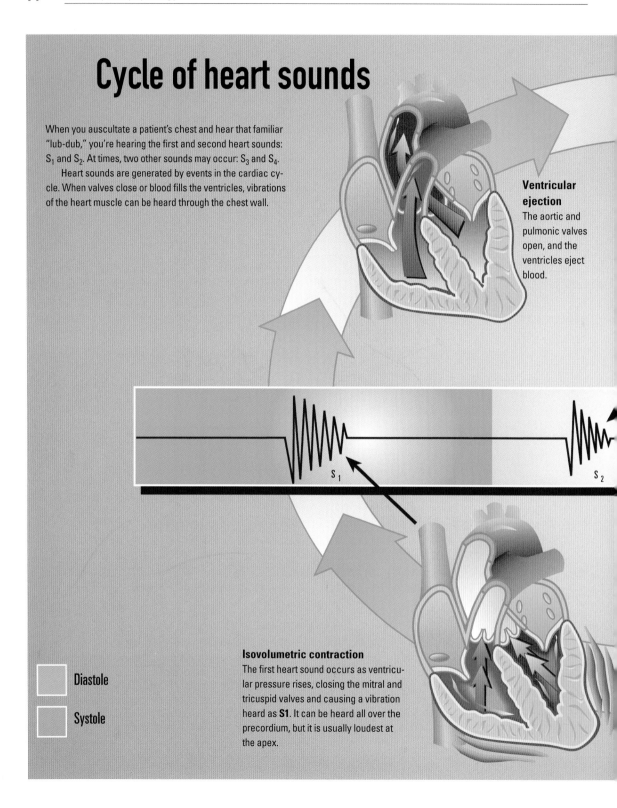

Ventricular ejection

The aortic and pulmonic valves open, and the ventricles eject blood.

S_1

S_2

Diastole

Systole

Isovolumetric contraction

The first heart sound occurs as ventricular pressure rises, closing the mitral and tricuspid valves and causing a vibration heard as **S1**. It can be heard all over the precordium, but it is usually loudest at the apex.

Isometric relaxation
The second heart sound occurs as ventricular pressure falls, and the aortic and pulmonic valves close, causing vibrations heard as **S2**. Although it is heard all over the precordium, it is loudest at the base.

Rapid ventricular filling
In some patients, ventricular filling causes vibrations heard as **S3**. However, normally this can be a silent event. In young adults, an S3 heart sound may be normal. An S3 heart sound is pathologic in patients with left-sided heart failure or mitral valve regurgitation. Since S3 is heard soon after S2, it is commonly referred to as a *ventricular gallop*.

S₃   S₄

Varying sound patterns
The phonogram at left shows how heart sounds vary in duration and intensity. For instance, S2 (which occurs when the semilunar valves snap shut) is a shorter-lasting sound than S1 because the semilunar valves take less time to close than the AV valves, which cause S1.

Slow ventricular filling
The fourth heart sound can occur at the end of diastole when the atria contract and eject blood into resistant ventricles, causing vibrations heard as **S4**. An S4 heart sound can be normal in older adults who do not have any evidence of heart disease. An S4 heart sound is pathologic in patients with aortic stenosis, coronary artery disease, cardiomyopathy, or left ventricular hypertrophy. Since the S4 heart sound can be heard just before S1, it is known as an *atrial gallop*.

Circulatory system

Arterial circulation

Blood flows through the arterial circulation in three types of vessels:

- *arteries* — have thick, muscular walls to accommodate high speed and pressure of blood flow

- *arterioles* — have thinner walls than arteries; control blood flow to capillaries
- *capillaries* — have microscopic walls composed of a single layer of endothelial cells.

Arteries can be classified according to their function:

- *Conductive arteries* typically have few branches and follow relatively straight lines. One example is the external iliac artery.
- *Distributive arteries* typically have multiple branches and arise from the conductive arteries.

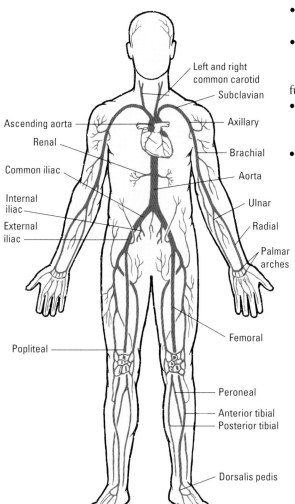

Left and right common carotid
Subclavian
Ascending aorta
Renal
Axillary
Common iliac
Brachial
Internal iliac
Aorta
External iliac
Ulnar
Radial
Palmar arches
Popliteal
Femoral
Peroneal
Anterior tibial
Posterior tibial
Dorsalis pedis

You think you're under pressure! Let me tell you what's going on in my world.

Venous circulation

Blood flows through the venous circulation in two types of vessels:

- *venules* — gather blood from the capillaries; have thinner walls than arterioles
- *veins* — have thinner walls but larger diameters than arteries because of the low pressure of venous return to the heart.

Changes in abdominal and thoracic pressures and pressure created by moving muscles keep blood moving toward the heart. Valves in the veins prevent blood backflow; most are located in smaller more distal veins. The largest vein, the vena cava, has no valves.

Path of circulation

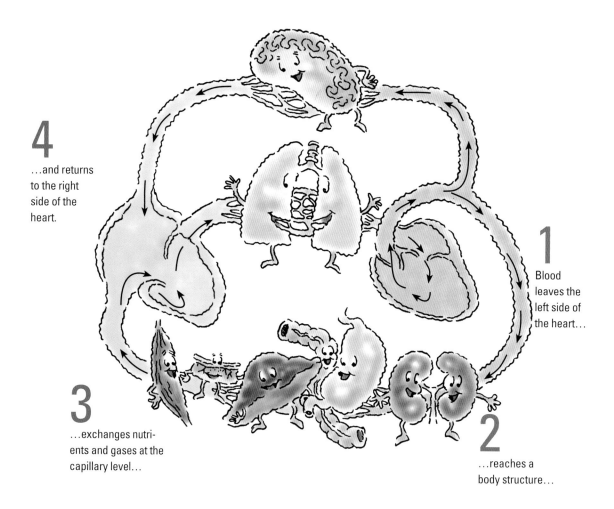

4 ...and returns to the right side of the heart.

1 Blood leaves the left side of the heart...

3 ...exchanges nutrients and gases at the capillary level...

2 ...reaches a body structure...

Specialized circulatory systems

The circulatory system involves more than the circulation of blood out of the heart. The heart muscle itself — as well as the brain, liver, and other organs — must receive a steady supply of oxygenated blood.

Circulation to the heart muscle

The heart relies on the coronary arteries and their branches for its supply of oxygenated blood. It also depends on the cardiac veins to remove oxygen-depleted blood.

During diastole, blood flows out of the heart and into the coronary arteries. The right coronary artery supplies blood to the right atrium, part of the left atrium, most of the right ventricle, and the inferior part of the left ventricle. The left coronary artery, which splits into the left anterior descending and circumflex arteries, supplies blood to the left atrium, most of the left ventricle, and most of the interventricular septum.

The cardiac veins lie superficial to the arteries. The largest vein, the coronary sinus, opens into the right atrium. Most of the major cardiac veins empty into the coronary sinus; the anterior cardiac veins, however, empty into the right atrium.

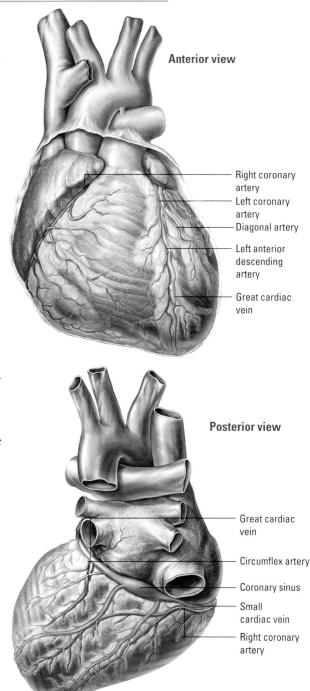

Anterior view

Right coronary artery
Left coronary artery
Diagonal artery
Left anterior descending artery
Great cardiac vein

Posterior view

Great cardiac vein
Circumflex artery
Coronary sinus
Small cardiac vein
Right coronary artery

Circulation to the brain

Four major arteries (the right and left carotid and the right and left vertebral arteries) supply the brain with oxygenated blood:

- The anterior brain is supplied with blood from the right and left internal carotid arteries. The right common carotid artery originates from the innominate artery, and the left common carotid artery arises directly from the aortic arch. These common carotid arteries branch in the neck into the internal carotid arteries, which enter the skull to deliver blood to the brain.
- The right and left vertebral arteries arise from the right and left subclavian arteries, course through the bony canal of the vertebrae, and converge to form the basilar artery. The basilar artery supplies blood to the posterior brain.

These four arteries join at the circle of Willis, an anastomosis at the base of the brain. A complete circle of Willis helps ensure that blood flow to the entire brain is maintained despite interruption of any one of the brain's major vessels.

Base of the brain

Left internal carotid artery

Circle of Willis

Basilar artery

Left vertebral artery

Circulation to the liver

Seventy-five percent of the blood in the liver comes from the portal vein that drains the GI tract. This blood is full of nutrients. The other 25% is oxygenated blood that comes from the hepatic artery.

Capillary beds form the sinusoids of the liver, where hepatocytes filter and store nutrients and toxins. The sinusoids empty into the hepatic vein for venous return to the heart.

The circulation of blood into and out of the liver figures prominently in some disease processes.

Able to label?

pulmonic valve

4.

right atrium

1. *tricuspid valve*

2. *right ventricle*

3.

left atrium

5.

Bicuspid valve 6.

left ventricle 7.

aortic valve

8.

Label the heart chambers and heart valves indicated on this illustration.

My word!

Unscramble the names of the five vessel types in the circulatory system. Then use the circled letters to answer the question posed.

Question: Which node is the heart's primary pacemaker?

1.   elvesun _v_ _e_ _(n)_ _v_ _(l)_ _e_ _s_

2.   areelsriot _(A)_ _r_ _(t)_ _e_ _r_ _(i)_ _o_ _l_ _e_ _s_

3.   siven _v_ _e_ _(i)_ _n_ _s_

4.   isacalliper _c_ _(a)_ _p_ _i_ _l_ _l_ _a_ _r_ _(i)_ _e_ _s_

5.   eatersir _a_ _(r)_ _t_ _e_ _r_ _(i)_ _s_

Answer: _s_ _i_ _n_ _o_ _a_ _t_ _r_ _i_ _a_ _l_

Suggested References

Copstead, L. Pathophysiology Text and Study Guide, 5th ed. St. Louis, MO: Elsevier Saunders, 2013.

Jarvis, C. Physical Examination & Health Assessment, 7th ed. St. Louis, MO: Elsevier Saunders, 2015.

Lewis, S.L., Dirksen, S.R., Heitkemper, M.M., & Bucher, L. Medical-Surgical Nursing: Assessment and Management of Clinical Problems, 9th ed. St. Louis, MO: Elsevier, 2014.

Answers: Able to label? 1. Right atrium, 2. Tricuspid valve, 3. Right ventricle, 4. Pulmonic valve, 5. Left atrium, 6. Mitral valve, 7. Left ventricle, 8. Aortic valve. My word! 1. Venules, 2. Arterioles, 3. Veins, 4. Capillaries, 5. Arteries; Question: Sinoatrial.

Chapter 2

Assessment

Taking a health history

The first step in assessing the cardiovascular system is to obtain a health history. Begin by introducing yourself and explaining what will occur during the health history and physical examination. Then, ask about the patient's chief complaint. Also, be sure to ask about both the patient's personal and family health history. Remember, the health history interview is an interview with a purpose.

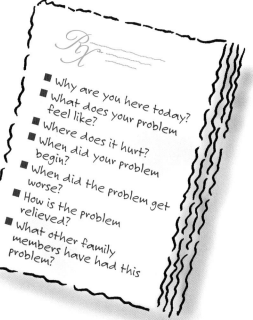

- Why are you here today?
- What does your problem feel like?
- Where does it hurt?
- When did your problem begin?
- When did the problem get worse?
- How is the problem relieved?
- What other family members have had this problem?

Common chief complaints

Angina (chest pain/chest discomfort)

Many patients with cardiovascular problems complain at some point of chest discomfort. Chest pain or discomfort can arise suddenly or gradually and can radiate to the arms, neck, jaw, or back. It can be steady or intermittent and mild or acute, and it can range in character from a sharp, shooting sensation to a feeling of heaviness, fullness, or even indigestion. The cause of chest pain or discomfort may be difficult to determine at first. It can be provoked or aggravated by stress, anxiety, exertion, deep breathing, or consumption of certain foods (http://www.heart.org/HEARTORG/Conditions/HeartAttack/DiagnosingaHeartAttack/Angina-Chest-Pain_UCM_450308_Article.jsp#.WQZe19y1uss).

> Steady or intermittent? Mild or acute? Sharp and shooting or heavy and full? Just trying to describe this chest pain is painful!

memory board
PQRST: What's the story?

Use the PQRST mnemonic to fully explore your patient's chest pain. When you ask the questions below, you'll encourage him/her to describe his/her symptom in greater detail.

***Remember to streamline your questions according to the patient's pain severity so that emergency care can be initiated promptly when indicated.**

Provocative or palliative	Quality or quantity	Region or radiation	Severity	Timing
» What provokes or relieves the chest pain? » What makes the pain worsen or subside?	» What does the pain feel like? » Are you having the pain right now? If so, is it more or less severe than usual? » To what degree does chest pain affect your normal activities?	» Where in the chest does the pain occur? » Does the pain appear in other regions as well? If so, where?	» How severe is the chest pain? How would you rate it on a scale of 0 to 10, with 10 being the most severe? » Does the pain seem to be diminishing, intensifying, or staying about the same?	» When did the pain begin? » Was the onset sudden or gradual? » How often does the pain occur? » How long does it last?

Palpitations

Defined as a conscious awareness of one's heartbeat, palpitations are usually felt over the precordium or in the throat or neck. Additionally, short circuits in the electrical conduction can lead to waves of abnormal firing (http://www.emedicinehealth.com/palpit ations/article_em.htm).

Palpitations may be regular or irregular, fast or slow, paroxysmal or sustained. Ask the patient to simulate his/her rhythm by tapping his/her finger on a hard surface.

Many palpitations are insignificant, and although oftentimes benign, palpitations are a symptom of a life-threatening arrhythmia (http://www.uptodate.com/contents/overview-of-palpitations-in-adults). They can be caused by disorders such as arrhythmias, hypertension, mitral prolapse, and mitral stenosis.

> *Rx*
> Ask the patient the following questions about his/her palpitations:
> - What are your palpitations like? For example, are they pounding, jumping, fluttering, or flopping or bopping?
> - Do you have a sensation of missed or skipped beats?
> - Do you have a history of hypertension?
> - Have you recently started digoxin therapy?
> - What medications do you take?
> - Do you smoke, drink caffeinated beverages, or consume alcohol? If so, how much?

> Are you sure that's what your palpitations feel like? That sounds an awful lot like "Jingle Bells."

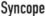

Syncope

Syncope is a brief, self-limiting loss of consciousness caused by a lack of blood to the brain. It usually occurs abruptly, is transient, lasting only seconds to minutes. Syncope may result from disorders such as aortic arch syndrome, aortic stenosis, acute myocardial infarction, aortic dissection, pulmonary embolus, and arrhythmias (Walsh, K., Hoffmayer, K., & Hamdan, M.H. Syncope: Diagnosis and Management. *Current Problems in Cardiology* 40(2):51–86, 2015).

Low flow states, some in association with CHF or advanced cardiomyopathy, may cause hypotension, resulting in transient cerebral hypoperfusion. When syncope occurs, the patient typically lies motionless, with his/her skeletal muscles relaxed. The depth of unconsciousness varies. The patient is strikingly pale with a slow, weak pulse; hypotension; and almost imperceptible breathing (http://emedicine.medscape.com/article/811669-overview#a8).

> *Rx*
> Ask the patient the following questions about his/her syncope:
> - Did you feel weak, light-headed, nauseous, or sweaty just before you fainted?
> - Did you get up quickly from a chair or from lying down?
> - During the fainting episode, did you have muscle spasms or incontinence?
> - How long were you unconscious?
> - When you regained consciousness, were you alert or confused? Did you have a headache?
> - Have you fainted before? If so, how often do the episodes occur?

> Hmm… He's pale and motionless; has a slow, weak pulse; and is hypotensive. He is barely breathing. I'd say he isn't getting enough blood to his/her brain.

Intermittent claudication

Intermittent claudication is severe, cramping limb pain that's brought on by exercise and relieved by 1 or 2 minutes of rest. It usually occurs in the legs and is the prominent symptom of peripheral arterial disease (PAD). This pain may be acute or chronic; when acute, it may signal acute arterial occlusion. Intermittent claudication typically results from disorders such as aortic arteriosclerotic occlusive disease, acute arterial occlusion, or arteriosclerosis obliterans (http://www.umm.edu/health/medical/reports/articles/peripheral-artery-disease-and-intermittent-claudication).

> Intermittent claudication really cramps my lifestyle.

Ask the patient the following questions about his/her intermittent claudication:
- How far can you walk before pain occurs?
- How long must you rest before it subsides?
- Can you walk as far as you could before, or must you rest more often?
- Does the pain-rest pattern vary?
- Has this symptom affected your lifestyle?

Peripheral edema

Peripheral edema results from excess interstitial fluid in the arms or legs. It may be unilateral or bilateral, slight or dramatic, and pitting or nonpitting. Arm edema may be caused by superior vena cava syndrome or thrombophlebitis. Leg edema may be an early sign of right-sided heart failure, thrombophlebitis, or chronic venous insufficiency.

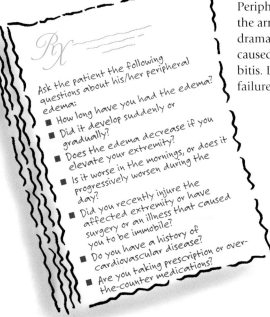

Ask the patient the following questions about his/her peripheral edema:
- How long have you had the edema?
- Did it develop suddenly or gradually?
- Does the edema decrease if you elevate your extremity?
- Is it worse in the mornings, or does it progressively worsen during the day?
- Did you recently injure the affected extremity or have surgery or an illness that caused you to be immobile?
- Do you have a history of cardiovascular disease?
- Are you taking prescription or over-the-counter medications?

Ask the patient with cardiovascular complaints if he or she has any of these signs or symptoms:
- shortness of breath on exertion, when lying down, or at night
- cough
- cyanosis or pallor
- weakness
- fatigue
- unexplained weight change
- dizziness
- headache
- high or low blood pressure
- peripheral skin changes, such as decreased hair distribution, skin color changes, or a thin, shiny appearance to the skin.

Other signs and symptoms

Ask the patient if he or she has any other signs or symptoms. Also, inquire about the patient's family history and past medical history, including history of heart disease, diabetes, or chronic lung, kidney, or liver disease.

Measuring blood pressure

Come equipped

When you take a patient's blood pressure, you're measuring the lateral force that blood exerts on the arterial walls as the heart contracts (systolic pressure) and relaxes (diastolic pressure). Use these tips to obtain the most accurate reading:

- Use a cuff that's 20% to 25% wider than the patient's arm circumference.
- Support the patient's arm at heart level.
- Use the bell of the stethoscope.
- Deflate the cuff at 2 to 3 mm Hg per second.
- Listen for the five phases of Korotkoff sounds.

Record the systolic blood pressure when you hear the first two consecutive sounds of phase I. With the onset of silence in phase V, record the diastolic pressure.

Systolic Korotkoff sounds
Phase I: Clear tapping sounds

Phase II: Tapping sounds with whooshing sounds

Phase III: Loud, high-pitched tapping sounds

First diastolic Korotkoff sound
Phase IV: Muffled sounds

Second diastolic Korotkoff sound
Phase V: Silence

Performing cardiac inspection

Take a moment to assess the patient's general appearance. Is he/ she overly thin? Obese? Alert? Anxious? Note the patient's skin color, temperature, turgor, and texture. Are his/her fingers clubbed? If the patient is dark skinned, inspect his/ her mucous membranes for pallor.

2

Next, inspect the chest. Note landmarks you can use to describe your findings and to identify structures underlying the chest wall. Also look for pulsations, symmetry of movement, retractions, or heaves (a strong outward thrust of the chest wall that occurs during systole).

3

Note the location of the apical impulse, including any displacement. You should find it in the fifth intercostal space, medial to the left midclavicular line. It's usually the point of maximal impulse (PMI) and can be seen in about 50% of adults. You'll notice it more easily in children and in patients with thin chest walls. Because the apical impulse corresponds to the apex of the heart, it helps indicate how well the left ventricle is working.

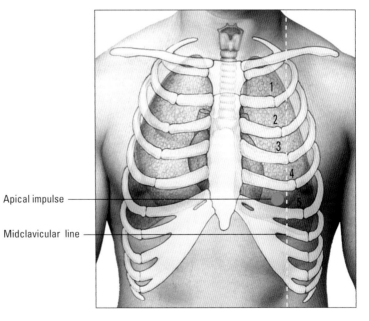

Apical impulse

Midclavicular line

Performing cardiac palpation and percussion

Maintain a gentle touch when you palpate so that you don't obscure pulsations or similar findings. Using the ball of your hand, then your fingertips, palpate over the precordium to find the apical impulse. Note heaves or thrills (fine vibrations that feel like the purring of a cat).

The apical impulse may be difficult to palpate in an obese or a pregnant patient and in a patient with a thick chest wall. If it's difficult to palpate with the patient lying on his/her back, have him/her lie on his/her left side or sit upright. It may also be helpful to have the patient exhale completely and hold his/her breath for a few seconds.

Follow the percussion map to help you find your way on your assessment journey. Listen closely, though, to make sure you're on the right path.

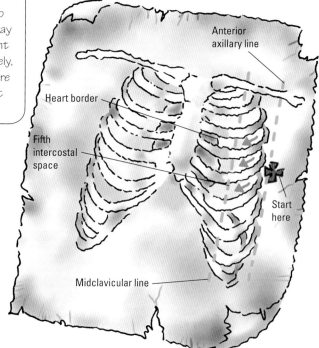

Anterior axillary line

Heart border

Fifth intercostal space

Start here

Midclavicular line

Begin percussing at the anterior axillary line, moving toward the sternum along the third, fourth, and fifth intercostal spaces. The sound changes from resonance to dullness over the left border of the heart, normally at the midclavicular line. The right border of the heart is usually aligned with the sternum and can't be percussed.

Auscultating for heart sounds

You can learn a great deal about the heart by auscultating for heart sounds.

Cardiac auscultation requires a methodical approach and lots of practice. Begin by identifying the four auscultation sites. Auscultation sites are identified by the names of heart valves but aren't located directly over the valves. Rather, these sites are located along the pathway blood takes as it flows through the heart's chambers and valves.

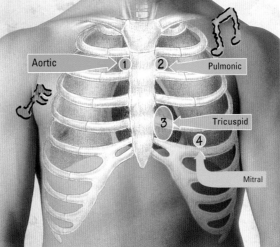

Aortic   ① ② Pulmonic

③ Tricuspid

④

Mitral

1

Begin auscultating over the **aortic area**, placing the stethoscope over the second intercostal space, along the right sternal border.

2

Then, move to the **pulmonic area**, located at the second intercostal space, at the left sternal border.

3

Next, assess the **tricuspid area**, which lies over the fourth and fifth intercostal spaces, along the left sternal border.

4

Finally, listen over the **mitral area**, located at the fifth intercostal space, near the midclavicular line.

Follow the site path

• In the **aortic area**, sounds reflect blood moving from the left ventricle during systole, crossing the aortic valve, and flowing through the aortic arch.
• In the **pulmonic area**, sounds reflect blood being ejected from the right ventricle during systole and then crossing the pulmonic valve and flowing through the main pulmonary artery.
• In the **tricuspid area**, sounds reflect movement of blood from the right atrium across the tricuspid valve and right ventricular filling during diastole.
• In the **mitral area**, also called the apical area, sounds reflect blood flow across the mitral valve and left ventricular filling during diastole.

Heart sounds

Systole is the period of ventricular contraction. As pressure in the ventricles increases, the mitral and tricuspid valves snap closed. That closure produces the first heart sound, S_1. At the end of ventricular contraction, the aortic and pulmonic valves snap shut. This produces the second heart sound, S_2.

Always identify S_1 and S_2 and then listen for adventitious sounds, such as third and fourth heart sounds (S_3 and S_4). Also listen for murmurs, which sound like vibrating, blowing, or rumbling noises.

To understand where extra heart sounds fall in relation to systole, diastole, and normal heart sounds, compare these illustrations.

Auscultation tips

• Concentrate as you listen for each sound.
• Avoid auscultating through clothing or wound dressings because these items can block sound.
• Avoid picking up extraneous sounds by keeping the stethoscope tubing off the patient's body and other surfaces.
• Until you become proficient at auscultation, explain to the patient that listening to his/her chest for a long period doesn't mean that anything is wrong.
• Ask the patient to breathe normally and to hold his/her breath periodically to enhance sounds that may be difficult to hear.

Identifying abnormal heart sounds

Murmurs

Cardiac murmurs are the result of turbulent blood flow (https://www.uptodate.com/contents/auscultation-of-cardiac-murmurs-in-adults). Murmurs can occur during systole or diastole and are described by several criteria. Their pitch can be high, medium, or low. They can vary in intensity or configuration, growing louder or softer. They can vary by location, sound pattern (blowing, harsh, or musical), radiation (to the neck or axillae), and period during which they occur in the cardiac cycle (pansystolic, midsystolic, or diastolic).

More on murmurs

If you identify a heart murmur, listen closely to determine its timing in the cardiac cycle. Then determine its other characteristics: quality (blowing, musical, harsh, or rumbling), pitch (medium, high, or low), and location (where the murmur sounds the loudest). Use a standard, six-level grading scale to describe the intensity (loudness) of the murmur.

Grade 1—barely audible, even to the trained ear
Grade 2—clearly audible
Grade 3—moderately loud
Grade 4—loud with palpable thrill
Grade 5—very loud with a palpable thrill; can be heard when the stethoscope has only partial contact with the chest
Grade 6—extremely loud with a palpable thrill; can be heard with the stethoscope lifted just off the chest wall

Photo op

The best way to hear murmurs is with the patient sitting up and leaning forward or lying on his/her left side, as shown at left. Listen for murmurs over the same precordial areas used in auscultation for heart sounds.

Murmur configurations

To help classify a murmur, begin by identifying its configuration (shape). Shown below are four basic patterns of murmurs.

Listen up! You can tell what's causing a murmur by how it sounds.

Crescendo/decrescendo
(diamond-shaped)
• Begins softly, peaks sharply, and then fades
• Examples: Pulmonic stenosis, aortic stenosis, mitral valve prolapse, mitral stenosis

Decrescendo
• Starts loudly and then gradually diminishes
• Examples: Aortic insufficiency, pulmonic insufficiency

Pansystolic
(holosystolic or plateau-shaped)
• Is uniform from beginning to end
• Examples: Mitral or tricuspid regurgitation

Crescendo
• Begins softly and then gradually increases
• Examples: Tricuspid stenosis, mitral valve prolapse

Differentiating murmurs

What you'll hear	Where you'll hear it	What causes it
• Medium pitch • Harsh quality • Possibly musical at apex • Loudest with expiration • Grade 4 or higher		Aortic stenosis
• Medium pitch • Harsh quality • Variable-grade intensity		Hypertrophic cardiomyopathy
• High pitch • Blowing quality • Grade 1 to 3 intensity		Aortic insufficiency
• Medium to high pitch • Blowing quality • Soft to loud grade intensity		Mitral insufficiency

What you'll hear	Where you'll hear it	What causes it
• Medium to high pitch • Blowing quality • Variable intensity • Increases slightly with inspiration		Tricuspid insufficiency
• High pitch • Harsh quality • Grade 5 or 6 intensity		Ventricular septal defect
• Low pitch • Rumbling quality • Grade 1 to 4 intensity		Mitral stenosis

○ = Bell

● = Diaphragm

Gallops and rubs

S_3: Classic sign of heart failure

S_3, also known as *ventricular gallop*, is commonly heard in children and may be normal in patients during the last trimester of pregnancy; however, it may be a cardinal sign of heart failure in older adults. Because it follows S_2, it's commonly compared to the "y" sound in "Ken-tuck-y." S_3 is low pitched; you'll hear it best at the apex when the patient is lying on his/her left side.

- In early ventricular diastole, the pulmonic and aortic valves snap closed, producing S_2.
- A large amount of blood rushes into the ventricles, possibly as a result of pulmonary edema, an atrial septal defect, or an acute myocardial infarction (MI).
- The rapid ventricular filling causes vibrations, producing S_3.

S_4: An MI aftereffect

Also called an *atrial gallop*, S_4 is an adventitious heart sound that you'll hear best over the tricuspid or mitral area when the patient lies on his/her left side. Patients who are elderly and those with hypertension, aortic stenosis, or a history of MI may have an S_4. It's commonly described as sounding like "Ten-nes-see" because it occurs just before S_1, after atrial contraction.

- In atrial diastole, the atria contract to eject blood into the ventricles.
- If the ventricles don't move or expand as much as they should, the atria must work harder to eject the blood. This causes the atria to vibrate, producing a sound known as S_4.
- As the ventricles fill and pressure rises, the mitral and tricuspid valves snap close, producing S_1.

Don't rub me the wrong way!

Listening for a pericardial friction rub is also an important part of your assessment. To do this, have the patient sit upright, lean forward, and exhale, as shown at left. Listen with the diaphragm of the stethoscope over the third intercostal space on the left side of the chest. A pericardial friction rub has a scratchy, rubbing quality. If you suspect a rub but have trouble hearing one, ask the patient to hold his/her breath.

Assessing the vascular system

Inspection

Start your assessment of the vascular system the same way you start an assessment of the cardiac system — by making general observations. For example, begin by examining the patient's arms when you take his/her vital signs. Complete your inspection by using the checklist at right.

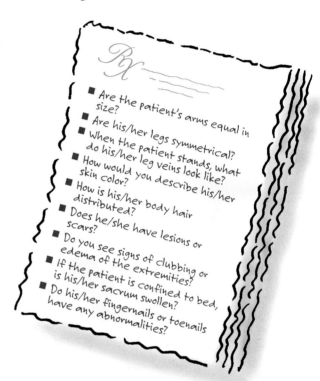

Rx

- Are the patient's arms equal in size?
- Are his/her legs symmetrical?
- When the patient stands, what do his/her leg veins look like?
- How would you describe his/her skin color?
- How is his/her body hair distributed?
- Does he/she have lesions or scars?
- Do you see signs of clubbing or edema of the extremities?
- If the patient is confined to bed, is his/her sacrum swollen?
- Do his/her fingernails or toenails have any abnormalities?

Assessing jugular vein distention

Now inspect the jugular veins. The internal jugular vein has a softer, undulating pulsation. Unlike the pulsation of the carotid artery, pulsation of the internal jugular vein changes in response to position, breathing, and palpation. The vein normally protrudes when the patient is lying down and lies flat when he or she stands.

When jugular vein distention is detected, place the patient at a 45-degree angle and then measure the distention with a horizontal straight edge aligned with the top of the pulsations. Then, read the vertical distance on a ruler. A measurement of 3 to 4 cm above the sternal angle is abnormal.

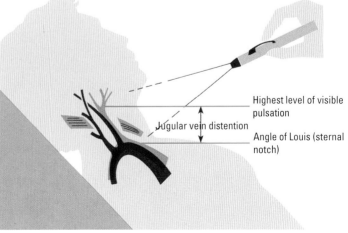

Highest level of visible pulsation

Jugular vein distention

Angle of Louis (sternal notch)

Palpation

The next step in an assessment of the vascular system is to palpate the arterial pulses. All pulses should be regular in rhythm and equal in strength.

To assess arterial pulses, apply pressure with your index and middle fingers.

Carotid pulse

Lightly place your fingers just medial to the trachea and below the jaw angle. Never *palpate both carotid arteries at the same time.*

Brachial pulse

Position your fingers medial to the biceps tendon.

Making the grade

Pulses are graded on the following scale:

4+   BOUNDING

3+   INCREASED

2+   NORMAL

1+   weak

0   ABSENT

Radial pulse

Apply gentle pressure to the medial and ventral side of the wrist, just below the base of the thumb.

A **HEAVE**, lifting of the chest wall felt during palpation along the left sternal border, may mean right ventricular hypertrophy; over the left ventricular area, a ventricular aneurysm.

A **THRILL**, which is a palpable vibration, usually suggests valvular dysfunction.

Dorsalis pedis pulse

Place your fingers on the medial dorsum of the foot while the patient points his/her toes down. The pulse is difficult to palpate here and may appear absent in a healthy patient.

Femoral pulse

Press relatively hard at a point inferior to the inguinal ligament. For an obese patient, palpate in the crease of the groin, halfway between the pubic bone and the hip bone.

Posterior tibial pulse

Apply pressure behind and slightly below the malleolus of the ankle.

Popliteal pulse

Press firmly in the popliteal fossa at the back of the knee.

Auscultation

Following the palpation sequence and using the bell of the stethoscope, listen over each artery. You shouldn't hear sounds over the carotid arteries. A bruit sounds like buzzing or blowing and could indicate arteriosclerotic plaque formation.

Assess the upper abdomen for abnormal pulsations, which could indicate the presence of an abdominal aortic aneurysm. Finally, auscultate the renal, iliac, femoral, and aortic pulses, checking for a bruit or other abnormal sounds.

Let's catch some waves!

To identify abnormal arterial pulses, check the waveforms below and see which one matches your patient's peripheral pulse.

Weak pulse

A weak pulse has a decreased amplitude with a slower upstroke and downstroke. Possible causes of a weak pulse include increased peripheral vascular resistance, as occurs in cold weather or with severe heart failure, and decreased stroke volume, as occurs with hypovolemia or aortic stenosis.

Bounding pulse

A bounding pulse has a sharp upstroke and downstroke with a pointed peak and elevated amplitude. Possible causes of bounding pulse include increased stroke volume, as with aortic insufficiency, or arterial wall stiffness, which can occur with aging.

Pulsus alternans

Pulsus alternans has a regular, alternating pattern of weak and strong pulses. This pulse is associated with left-sided heart failure.

Pulsus bigeminus

Pulsus bigeminus is similar to pulsus alternans but occurs at irregular intervals. This pulse is caused by premature atrial or ventricular beats.

Pulsus paradoxus

Pulsus paradoxus has increases and decreases in amplitude associated with the respiratory cycle. Marked decreases occur when the patient inhales. Pulsus paradoxus is associated with pericardial tamponade, advanced heart failure, and constrictive pericarditis.

Inspiration   Expiration

Pulsus bisferiens

Pulsus bisferiens shows an initial upstroke, a subsequent downstroke, and then another upstroke during systole. Pulsus bisferiens is caused by aortic stenosis and aortic insufficiency.

Abdominal auscultation points

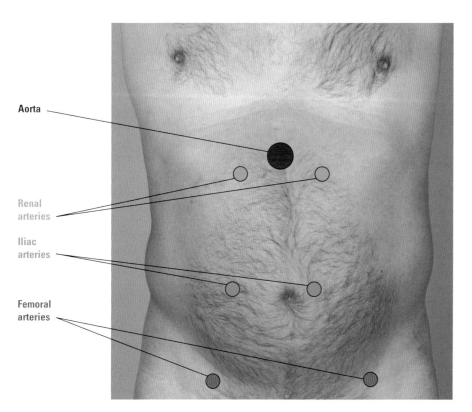

Aorta

Renal
arteries

Iliac
arteries

Femoral
arteries

What's all the bruit ha ha?
When auscultating over an artery, you may hear a bruit — a vascular sound similar to a heart murmur that may be caused by turbulent blood flow through a narrowed artery. Occasionally, you may hear a bruit limited to systole in the epigastric region of a healthy person.

Identifying abnormal vascular findings

If a patient has nonpitting edema in an extremity, measure the circumference of the affected and unaffected limbs and compare the difference. Take measurements regularly to detect changes.

Peripheral edema

Edema (swelling) may indicate heart failure or venous insufficiency. It may also be caused by varicosities or thrombophlebitis.

Pitting edema is swelling, usually of venous origin that results in a pit or depression in the affected area when a thumb is pressed firmly, but gently, into the skin for at least 5 seconds. Swelling caused primarily by lymph fluid collection in a dependent area may not cause pitting.

It's the pits!

Pitting edema is graded on a four-point scale.

0 = no pitting although edema may be present
+1 = 2 mm indentation
+2 = 4 mm indentation
+3 = 6 mm indentation
+4 = 8 mm indentation

Vascular insufficiency

Assessment findings differ in patients with arterial insufficiency and those with chronic venous insufficiency.

Arterial insufficiency

Pale, cool, shiny skin

Decreased or absent pulses

Deep red skin when extremity is dependent

Ulcers around toes

Thick, ridged nails

Chronic venous insufficiency

Pitting edema

Brown pigment

Difficult-to-find pulses (because of edema)

Ulcers around ankle

Cyanosis when extremity is dependent

Matchmaker

Match the murmur configuration shown with the name that describes it.

1. A. Decrescendo

2. B. Crescendo

3. C. Pansystolic

4. D. Crescendo/decrescendo

Able to label?

Identify the signs and symptoms of arterial insufficiency indicated on this illustration.

1.
2.
3.
4.
5.

Answers: Matchmaker 1. D, 2. A, 3. C, 4. B; Able to label? 1. Pale, shiny skin, 2. Decreased pulses, 3. Redness, 4. Ulcer, 5. Thick, rigid nails.

Suggested References

http://www.heart.org/HEARTORG/Conditions/HeartAttack/DiagnosingaHeartAttack/Angina-Chest-Pain_UCM_450308_Article.jsp#.WQZe19y1uss

Walsh, K., Hoffmayer, K., & Hamdan, M.H. Syncope: Diagnosis and Management, *Current Problems in Cardiology* 40(2):51–86, 2015.

Chapter 3

Diagnostic tests

Blood tests

Tests to identify myocardial infarction

After a myocardial infarction (MI), damaged cardiac tissue releases significant amounts of enzymes and proteins into the blood. Specific blood tests help confirm the diagnosis of MI, reveal the extent of cardiac damage, help monitor the healing progress, and assess reperfusion after the use of fibrinolytics.

Some blood tests, such as cardiac enzyme and protein tests, evaluate damage to the heart muscle. Other tests help to identify patients at risk for heart disease.

Serum cardiac biomarkers

- Myoglobin
  - Elevated
  - First marker of cardiac injury after acute MI
  - Found in skeletal muscle
- Creatine kinase (CK) and CK-MB
  - Both return to normal quickly
  - CK-MB most reliable when reported as a percentage of total CK (relative index)
  - Found in cardiac muscle (CK-MB) and skeletal muscle (CK)
  Troponin I and troponin T are myocardial regulatory proteins that control the calcium-mediated interaction of actin and myosin (Adams, Abendschein, & Jaffe, 1993).
- Troponin I
  - Isotype of troponin found only in myocardium
  - Elevated
  - Specific to myocardial damage
- Troponin T
  - Isotype of troponin that's less specific to myocardial damage (can indicate renal failure)
  - Elevated
  - Determined quickly at bedside

Values

Myoglobin

- Normal value: 0 to 0.09 mcg/ml
- Rises within 30 minutes to 4 hours
- Peaks within 6 to 10 hours
- Returns to baseline by 24 hours

CK-MB

- Normal value: 38 to 190 units/L for men; 10 to 150 units/L for women
- Rises within 4 to 8 hours
- Peaks in 12 to 24 hours
- May remain elevated for up to 96 hours

Troponin I

- Normal value: Less than 0.4 mcg/ml (may vary depending on the laboratory)
- Rises within 4 to 6 hours
- Peaks in 12 hours
- Returns to baseline in 3 to 10 days

Troponin T

- Normal value: Less than 0.1 mcg/ml (may vary depending on the laboratory)
- Rises within 4 to 8 hours
- Peaks in 12 to 48 hours
- Returns to baseline in 7 to 10 days

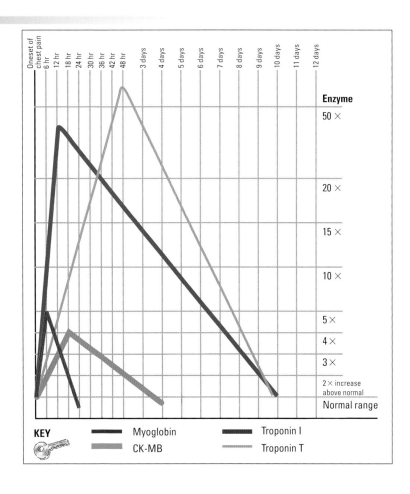

Tests to identify the risk of heart disease

Homocysteine (tHcy)

- Normal value: ≤13 µmol/L
- Excess levels
  - Irritate blood vessels, leading to atherosclerosis
  - Raise low-density lipoprotein (LDL) levels
  - Make blood clot more easily

High-sensitivity C-reactive protein (hs-CRP)

- Normal value: 0.1 to 0.3 mg/dl
- Excess levels: May indicate increased risk of coronary artery disease (CAD)

Triglycerides

- Normal value: <150 mg/dl
- Excess levels: Help with early identification of hyperlipidemia and identification of patients at risk for CAD

Total cholesterol

- Normal value: <200 mg/dl for adults; <170 mg/dl for children and adolescents
- Excess levels: May indicate hereditary lipid disorders, CAD

Evaluating lipid test results

Use this chart to determine an adult patient's risk of CAD.

Lipoprotein fractionation

Lipoprotein fractionation tests isolate and measure high-density lipoproteins (HDLs), LDLs, and very-low-density lipoproteins (VLDLs). Each of these particles is composed of protein, cholesterol, and triglyceride in varying amounts.

HDL
- Primarily protein
- Test measures the actual amount in the blood
- The *higher* the level, the *lower* the risk of CAD
- Normal values for males, 35 to 65 mg/dl; for females, 35 to 80 mg/dl

LDL
- Mainly cholesterol
- Equal to total cholesterol—HDL cholesterol—VLDL cholesterol (when triglyceride level is below 400 mg/dl)
- The *higher* the LDL level, the *higher* the risk of CAD
- Normal levels for individuals without CAD, <130 mg/dl
- Optimal levels for individuals with CAD, <100 mg/dl

VLDL
- Mainly triglycerides
- Calculated as triglyceride level ÷ 5
- The *higher* the VLDL level, the *higher* the risk of CAD
- Can be measured with a more sensitive test when high-risk patients and those with triglyceride levels of 400 mg/dl or more require complex medical management

Tests to identify the risk of heart failure

Heart cells produce and store two neurohormones — A-type natriuretic peptide (ANP) and B-type natriuretic peptide (BNP) — that help ensure cardiac equilibrium. Disruptions in fluid balance within the circulatory system trigger release of these hormones, which act as natural diuretics and antihypertensives.

ANP

- Found in atrial tissue
- Normal value: 20 to 77 pg/ml

BNP

- Found in ventricular tissue
- Helps accurately diagnose and grade heart failure severity
- Normal value: <100 pg/ml

ANP is released by the atria in response to acute increased fluid volume and pressure.

The atria and ventricles become enlarged in response to increased fluid volume.

BNP is released by the ventricles in response to prolonged fluid volume overload or elevated pressure.

Correlating the degree of heart failure with BNP level

The higher a patient's level of BNP, the greater the degree of heart failure. In turn, the greater the degree of heart failure, the more the patient's ability to perform activities of daily living (ADLs) will be impaired. Use this chart to help you plan your nursing care.

New York Heart Association Classification

IV: Severe to complete limitation of ADLs

III: Marked limitation of ADLs

II: Slight limitation of ADLs

I: No limitation of ADLs

0: Normal

0   500   1000   1500

BNP in pg/ml

Tests for general screening

General screening tests are used to evaluate overall health and response to treatment.

Electrolyte tests

Electrolytes — which occur in the fluids both inside and outside cells — are crucial for nearly all cellular reactions and functions.

Potassium, calcium, magnesium

Sodium, chloride, carbon dioxide

▲ Potassium
• Most critical value
• Has narrow therapeutic range
• Imbalances cause life-threatening arrhythmias
• Affected by diuretics, penicillin G, some nonsteroidal anti-inflammatory drugs

● Calcium
• High values cause cardiac toxicity and arrhythmias
• Elevations commonly caused by cancer, kidney disease, and hyperparathyroidism (http://www.healthline.com/health/electrolyte-disorders#types4)

■ Magnesium
• High values cause ECG changes, ventricular tachycardia, and ventricular fibrillation
• Low values cause ECG changes, bradycardia, and hypotension

Sodium
• Maintains osmotic pressure, acid-base balance, and nerve impulse transmission
• Levels decreased in severe heart failure
• Decreased by diuretics, high triglycerides, and low blood protein

Chloride
• Partners with sodium to maintain fluid and acid-base balance
• Low levels in heart failure and metabolic acidosis

Carbon dioxide
• Primarily made up of bicarbonate
• Regulated by the kidneys
• Levels lowered by thiazide diuretics

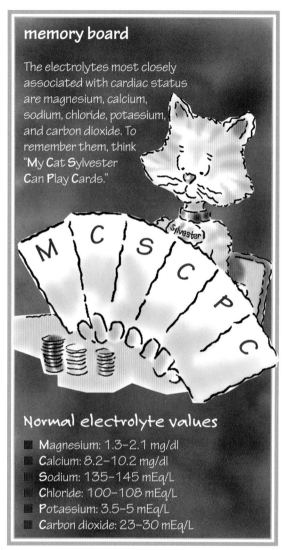

memory board

The electrolytes most closely associated with cardiac status are magnesium, calcium, sodium, chloride, potassium, and carbon dioxide. To remember them, think "My Cat Sylvester Can Play Cards."

Normal electrolyte values
■ Magnesium: 1.3–2.1 mg/dl
■ Calcium: 8.2–10.2 mg/dl
▥ Sodium: 135–145 mEq/L
▥ Chloride: 100–108 mEq/L
■ Potassium: 3.5–5 mEq/L
■ Carbon dioxide: 23–30 mEq/L

Coagulation tests

Activated partial thromboplastin time (aPTT), prothrombin time (PT), bleeding time, and activated clotting time (ACT) are tests that measure clotting time. They're used to measure response to treatment as well as to screen for clotting disorders.

Understanding clotting

Clotting is initiated through two different pathways.

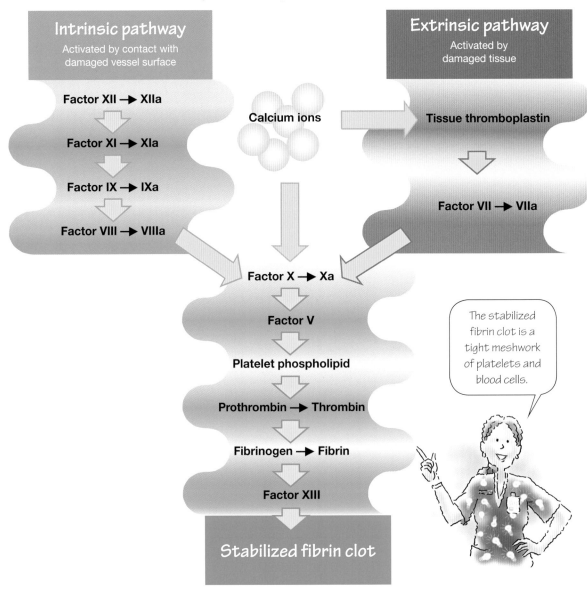

Common tests for clotting

Test	Action	Clinical uses	Location performed	Normal range	Therapeutic ranges	Panic value
ACT	Measures overall coagulation activity	♥ Evaluates effects of high-dose heparin therapy during cardiac procedures	Bedside	70 to 120 seconds	2 times normal range	Unknown
Bleeding time	Determines platelet function abnormalities	♥ Screens for platelet abnormalities before or during surgery ♥ Used to diagnose von Willebrand's disease, vascular disorders, hemostatic dysfunctions	Bedside	3 to 10 minutes	Unknown	>15 minutes
aPTT	Measures defects in intrinsic and common clotting pathways	♥ Evaluates effects of heparin therapy ♥ Assesses overall coagulation system	Laboratory	21 to 35 seconds	2 to 2.5 times normal range	>70 seconds
PT	Directly measures deficits in extrinsic and common clotting pathways	♥ Evaluates effects of coumarin therapies ♥ Assesses for vitamin K deficiency ♥ Used to diagnose liver failure	Laboratory	11 to 13 seconds	2 to 2.5 times normal range	>30 seconds

Understanding INR

Because PT measurements vary from laboratory to laboratory, international normalized ratio (INR) is generally viewed as the best standardized measurement of PT. Both are used for monitoring warfarin treatment. Guidelines for patients receiving warfarin therapy recommend an INR of 2.0 to 3.0, except for patients with mechanical prosthetic heart valves. For those patients, an INR of 2.5 to 3.5 is recommended.

What's the problem?

When the INR is higher than the recommended range, it means that your blood clots more slowly than desired, and a lower INR means your blood clots more quickly than desired (http://www.mayoclinic.org/tests-procedures/prothrombin-time/details/results/rsc-20163828).

Increased INR values may indicate disseminated intravascular coagulation, cirrhosis, hepatitis, vitamin K deficiency, salicylate intoxication, or uncontrolled oral anticoagulation.

Electrocardiography

12-lead ECG

A commonly used diagnostic tool, the 12-lead ECG can help identify myocardial ischemia, MI, rhythm and conduction disturbances, chamber enlargement, electrolyte imbalances, and drug toxicity. The standard 12-lead ECG uses a series of electrodes placed on the patient's extremities and chest wall to assess the heart from 12 different views (leads).

Six unipolar precordial leads (V_1 to V_6) show the heart from the **horizontal plane**.

Three bipolar limb leads (I, II, and III) and three unipolar augmented limb leads (aV_R, aV_L, and aV_F) show the heart from the **frontal plane**.

Ground

Understanding ECG leads

ECG waveforms vary depending on the leads being viewed and the rhythm of the heart. To make an accurate assessment of the heart's electrical activity, an ECG needs to be evaluated from every view.

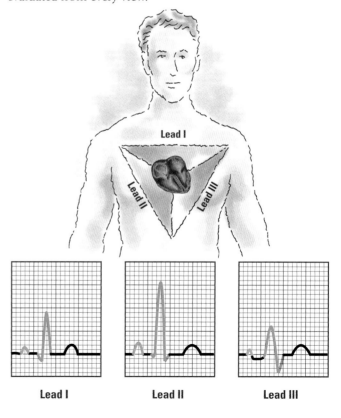

Lead I

Lead II

Lead III

Lead I   **Lead II**   **Lead III**

Locating myocardial damage with a 12-lead ECG

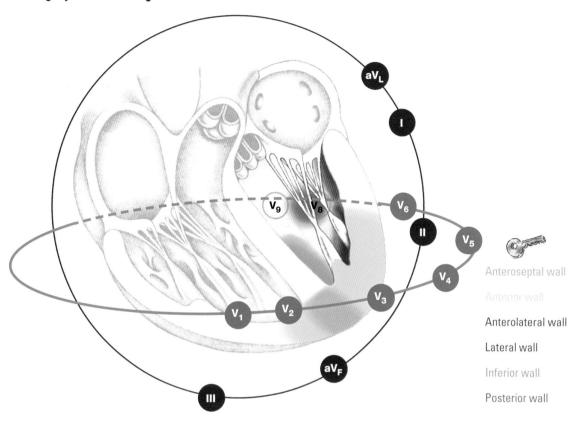

Anteroseptal wall

Anterior wall

Anterolateral wall

Lateral wall

Inferior wall

Posterior wall

Wall affected	Leads	Artery involved	Reciprocal changes
Anteroseptal	V_1, V_2, V_3, V_4	Left anterior descending (LAD)	None
Anterior	V_2, V_3, V_4	Left coronary artery (LCA) and LAD	II, III, aV_F
Anterolateral	I, aV_L, V_3, V_4, V_5, V_6	LAD and diagonal branches, circumflex and marginal branches	II, III, aV_F
Lateral	I, aV_L, V_5, V_6	Circumflex branch of LCA	II, III, aV_F
Inferior	II, III, aV_F	Right coronary artery (RCA)	I, aV_L
Posterior	V_8, V_9	RCA or circumflex	V_1, V_2, V_3, V_4 (R greater than S in V_1 and V_2, ST-segment depression, elevated T wave)

Right precordial ECG lead placement

A right-sided ECG provides information about the extent of damage to the right ventricle, especially during the first 12 hours of an MI. The leads used to obtain a right-sided ECG, called the *right precordial leads*, are designated by the letter "V," a number representing the electrode position, and the letter "R," which indicates placement on the right side of the chest. To record the right precordial chest leads, place the electrodes as follows:

- V_1R — fourth intercostal space (ICS), left sternal border
- V_2R — fourth ICS, right sternal border
- V_3R — halfway between V_2R and V_4R
- V_4R — fifth ICS, right midclavicular line
- V_5R — fifth ICS, right anterior axillary line
- V_6R — fifth ICS, right midaxillary line

Midclavicular line
Anterior axillary line
Midaxillary line

Damage to the right ventricle commonly results from occlusion of the right coronary artery.

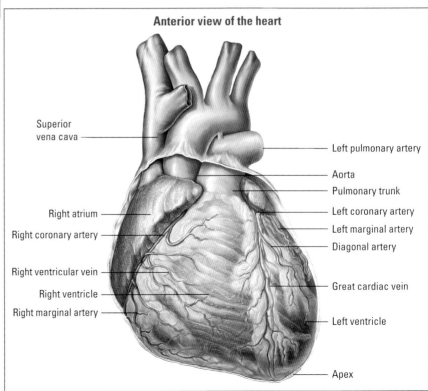

Anterior view of the heart

Superior vena cava

Left pulmonary artery

Aorta
Pulmonary trunk
Left coronary artery

Right atrium

Left marginal artery

Right coronary artery

Diagonal artery

Right ventricular vein

Great cardiac vein

Right ventricle

Right marginal artery

Left ventricle

Apex

Posterior ECG lead placement

Because of lung and muscle barriers, the usual precordial chest leads can't "see" the heart's posterior surface to record myocardial damage in this area. To assess the posterior heart, some practitioners add three posterior leads to the standard 12-lead ECG. These leads are designated as V_7, V_8, and V_9.

To ensure an accurate reading, make sure the posterior electrodes are placed at the same horizontal level as V_6, at the fifth intercostal space. Place lead V_7 at the posterior axillary line, lead V_9 at the paraspinal line, and lead V_8 halfway between leads V_7 and V_9.

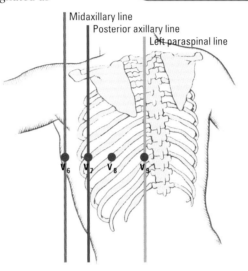

Midaxillary line
Posterior axillary line
Left paraspinal line

V_6 V_7 V_8 V_9

Posterior view of heart

- Superior vena cava
- Aortic arch
- Right pulmonary artery
- Left atrium
- Right pulmonary veins
- Right atrium
- Inferior vena cava
- Small cardiac vein
- Right coronary artery
- Coronary sinus
- Middle cardiac veins
- Right ventricle

Left pulmonary artery
Left pulmonary veins
Great cardiac vein
Circumflex artery
Left posterior ventricular artery branches
Left posterior ventricular vein
Left ventricle

Damage to the posterior walls can result from occlusion of the right coronary or left circumflex arteries.

Exercise ECG

Exercise ECG, or *stress testing*, is a noninvasive procedure that helps assess the heart's response to an increased workload. Continuous ECG monitoring is used to record the heart's electrical activity while the patient performs a standardized exercise protocol. Stop the test if the patient experiences chest pain, fatigue, severe dyspnea, claudication, weakness or dizziness, hypotension, pallor or vasoconstriction, disorientation, ataxia, ischemic ECG changes, rhythm disturbances or heart block, or ventricular conduction abnormalities.

Drug-induced stress tests

If a patient can't tolerate physical activity, a drug (dipyridamole, adenosine, or dobutamine) can be administered to cause the heart to react as if the person were exercising. The drug is given I.V. along with a radioactive substance known as a *tracer*. Those areas of the heart muscle that lack adequate blood supply pick up the tracer very slowly, if at all.

A nuclear scanner records a set of images; a second set of images is taken 30 minutes to 3 hours later. A cardiologist uses these images to determine areas of heart muscle with diminished blood supply or permanent damage from an MI.

Holter monitoring

Also called *ambulatory ECG*, Holter monitoring records the heart's activity as the patient follows his or her normal routine. The patient wears a small electronic recorder connected to electrodes placed on the chest and keeps a diary of his or her activities and associated symptoms. Used to identify intermittent arrhythmias, this test usually lasts about 24 hours.

A look at a Holter monitor

Portable ECG recorder

Patient event marker button

ECG leadwires

Patient Holter monitor log

| 7/5/10 | 15:30 | I was doing the laundry. Suddenly, my heart was racing and I felt weak. |

Electrophysiology studies

Electrophysiology studies are used to help determine the cause of an arrhythmia and the best treatment for it. A bipolar or tripolar electrode catheter is threaded into a vein, through the right atrium, and across the septal leaflet of the tricuspid valve. The heart's usual conduction is recorded first. The catheter sends electrical signals to the heart to change the heart rate and initiate an arrhythmia. Various drugs are then tried to terminate the arrhythmia.

The femoral vein is the most common choice for catheter insertion. However, the subclavian, internal jugular, or brachial vein may also be used.

Femoral vein

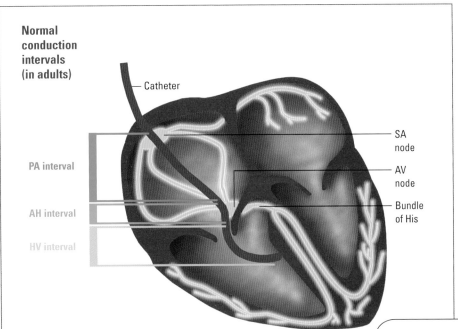

Normal conduction intervals (in adults)

Catheter

SA node

AV node

Bundle of His

PA interval

AH interval

HV interval

PA interval = conduction from SA node to AV node = 20 to 40 msec
AH interval = conduction from AV node to bundle of His = 45 to 150 msec
HV interval = conduction from bundle of His to ventricles = 35 to 55 msec

Sometimes the cardiologist can induce an arrhythmia and then immediately treat it using radiofrequency ablation, a pacemaker, or an implantable cardioverter-defibrillator.

Imaging tests

Various imaging and radiographic tests are used to help visualize heart structures and blood vessels throughout the cardiovascular system. Although many of these tests are noninvasive and quick to perform, some require the insertion of a cardiac catheter, injection of a contrast medium, or nuclear medicine to further enhance the view.

Cardiac catheterization

Cardiac catheterization involves passing a catheter through veins and arteries to perform various measurements. It's used to:
- measure heart chamber and pulmonary artery pressures
- check blood flow between the heart chambers
- determine valve competence
- monitor cardiac wall contractility
- detect intracardiac shunts
- visualize the coronary arteries.

Right-sided heart catheterization

Superior vena cava
Pulmonary artery
Right atrium
Right ventricle
Brachial vein
Inferior vena cava
Femoral vein

Upper limits of normal pressure curves

Chambers of the right side of the heart
Two pressure complexes are represented for each chamber. Complexes at the far right in this diagram represent simultaneous recordings of pressures from the right atrium, right ventricle, and pulmonary artery.

Pressure (mm Hg)

RA = Right atrium
RV = Right ventricle
PA = Pulmonary artery
a wave = Contraction
v wave = Passive filling
1 = RV peak systolic pressure
2 = RV end-diastolic pressure
3 = PA peak systolic pressure
4 = PA dicrotic notch
5 = PA diastolic pressure

Now just because the cardiac cath showed you have an incompetent valve doesn't mean you aren't qualified for your job.

Chambers of the left side of the heart

Overall pressure configurations in the left side of the heart are similar to those of the right side of the heart, but pressures are significantly higher because systemic flow resistance is much greater than pulmonary resistance.

Pressure (mm Hg)

Left-sided heart catheterization

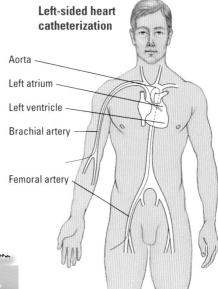

Aorta

Left atrium

Left ventricle

Brachial artery

Femoral artery

Bumpy road ahead

LA = Left atrium
LV = Left ventricle
Asc Ao = Ascending aorta
a wave = Contraction
v wave = Passive filling
1 = LV peak systolic pressure
2 = LV end-diastolic pressure
3 = PA peak systolic pressure
4 = PA dicrotic notch
5 = PA diastolic pressure

Watch your patient for bradycardia, hypotension, and nausea during femoral catheter removal.

Echocardiography

An echocardiograph uses ultra-high-frequency sound waves to help examine the size, shape, and motion of the heart's structures. Here's how it works.

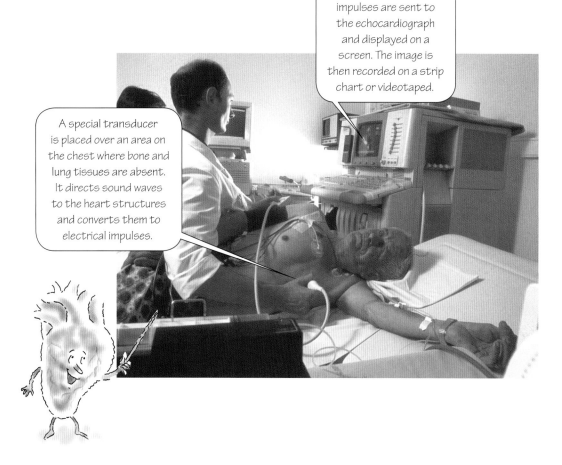

> These electrical impulses are sent to the echocardiograph and displayed on a screen. The image is then recorded on a strip chart or videotaped.

> A special transducer is placed over an area on the chest where bone and lung tissues are absent. It directs sound waves to the heart structures and converts them to electrical impulses.

Picture this!

This computer graphic depicts an image of the heart's chambers and valves that's more detailed than an X-ray. The ultrasound waves that rebound (or echo) off the heart can show the size, shape, and movement of cardiac structures as well as the flow of blood through the heart, which helps analyze valvular function and heart pressures.

Comparing two types of echocardiography

The most commonly used echocardiographic techniques are M-mode (motion mode) and two-dimensional. In many cases, the techniques are performed together to complement each other. Echocardiography may be used to detect mitral stenosis, mitral valve prolapse, aortic insufficiency, wall motion abnormalities, and pericardial effusion. The shaded areas beneath the transducer identify cardiac structures that intercept and reflect the transducer's ultrasonic waves.

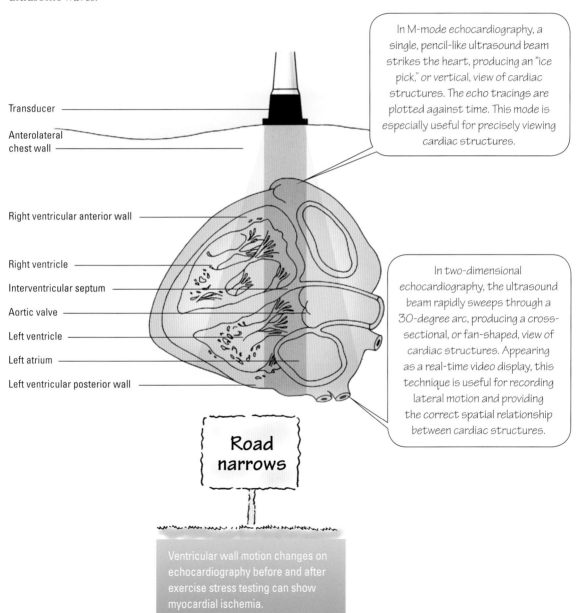

In M-mode echocardiography, a single, pencil-like ultrasound beam strikes the heart, producing an "ice pick," or vertical, view of cardiac structures. The echo tracings are plotted against time. This mode is especially useful for precisely viewing cardiac structures.

Transducer

Anterolateral chest wall

Right ventricular anterior wall

Right ventricle

Interventricular septum

Aortic valve

Left ventricle

Left atrium

Left ventricular posterior wall

In two-dimensional echocardiography, the ultrasound beam rapidly sweeps through a 30-degree arc, producing a cross-sectional, or fan-shaped, view of cardiac structures. Appearing as a real-time video display, this technique is useful for recording lateral motion and providing the correct spatial relationship between cardiac structures.

Road narrows

Ventricular wall motion changes on echocardiography before and after exercise stress testing can show myocardial ischemia.

Transesophageal echocardiography

In transesophageal echocardiography (TEE), ultrasonography is combined with endoscopy to provide a better view of the heart's structures.

How it's done

A small transducer is attached to the end of a gastroscope and inserted into the esophagus so that images of the heart's structure can be taken from the posterior of the heart. This test causes less tissue penetration and interference from chest wall structures and produces high-quality images of the thoracic aorta (except for the superior ascending aorta, which is shadowed by the trachea).

It must be TEE time!

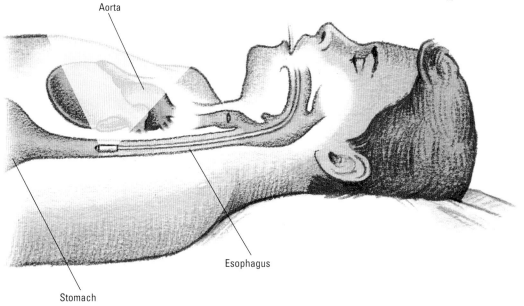

Aorta

Esophagus

Stomach

And why

The detailed pictures provided by TEE can help doctors see:

- the size of your heart and how thick its walls are
- how well your heart is pumping
- if there is abnormal tissue around your heart valves that could indicate bacterial, viral, or fungal infections or cancer
- if blood is leaking backward through your heart valves (regurgitation) or if your valves are narrowed or blocked (stenosis)
- if blood clots are in the chambers of your heart, in particular the upper chamber, for example, after a stroke. http://www.heart.org/HEARTORG/Conditions/HeartAttack/DiagnosingaHeartAttack/Transesophageal-Echocardiography TEE_UCM_441655_Article.jsp#.WYeJfFGQyss

TEE is used to evaluate valvular disease or repairs. It's also used to diagnose:

- thoracic and aortic disorders
- endocarditis
- congenital heart disease
- intracardiac thrombi
- tumors.

memory board

Complications of TEE

Respiratory depression from sedation
Aspiration of secretions into the trachea
Vasovagal reaction from vagus nerve stimulation
Esophageal perforation by transducer (watch for increased swallowing by the patient)

Cardiac magnetic resonance imaging

Also known as *nuclear magnetic resonance*, cardiac magnetic resonance imaging (MRI) yields high-resolution, tomographic, three-dimensional images of the heart. Cardiac MRI permits visualization of valve leaflets and structures, pericardial abnormalities and processes, ventricular hypertrophy, cardiac neoplasm, infarcted tissue, anatomic malformations, and structural deformities. It can be used to monitor the progression of ischemic heart disease and the effectiveness of treatment.

The MRI scanner records the electromagnetic signals the nuclei emit. The scanner then translates the signals into detailed pictures. The resulting images show tissue characteristics without lung or bone interference, as shown here.

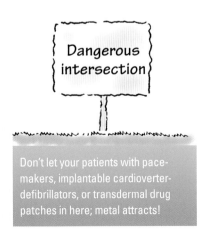

Dangerous intersection

Don't let your patients with pacemakers, implantable cardioverter-defibrillators, or transdermal drug patches in here; metal attracts!

Cardiac positron emission tomography

Cardiac positron emission tomography (PET) scanning combines elements of computed tomography scanning and conventional radionuclide imaging.

How it works

You can reassure your patient undergoing PET that he's getting no more radiation than a routine X-ray — but much better pictures.

1 Radioisotopes are administered to the patient by injection, inhalation, or I.V. infusion. One isotope targets blood; one targets glucose.

2 These isotopes emit particles called *positrons*.

3 The PET scanner detects and reconstructs the positrons to form an image.

What it shows

- Normal blood flow and glucose metabolism indicates good coronary perfusion.
- Decreased blood flow with increased glucose metabolism indicates ischemia.
- Decreased blood flow with decreased glucose metabolism shows necrotic or scarred heart tissue.

Cardiac blood pool imaging (wall motion study)

Cardiac blood pool imaging (also called *multiple-gated acquisition [MUGA] scanning*) is used to evaluate regional and global ventricular performance or the heart's pumping function, specifically the left ventricle.

https://www.unitypoint.org/cedarrapids/filesimages/Physician%20 and%20Clinics/Cardiology/Patient%20ed%202016/UPC_Cardiac%20 Blood%20Pool_5-13.pdf

During a MUGA scan, the camera records 14 to 64 points of a single cardiac cycle, yielding sequential images that can be studied like a motion picture film. This allows doctors to evaluate regional wall motion and determine ejection fraction and other indices of cardiac function.

Varieties are the spice of life

Many variations of the MUGA scan are available:
• In the *stress MUGA* test, the same test is performed at rest and after exercise to detect changes in ejection fraction and cardiac output.
• In the *nitroglycerin MUGA* test, the scintillation camera records points in the cardiac cycle after the sublingual administration of nitroglycerin to assess the drug's effect on ventricular function.

Blood flow

I love being the star of the show! Do you think this picture does me justice?

Did you know?

The MUGA scan is the most accurate way to measure ejection fraction? On-cologists use it to detect early signs of heart damage from cardiotoxic chemo-therapeutic drugs such as doxorubicin hydrochloride (Doxil).

Hot and cold spot imaging

^{99m}Tc + MI = HOT

Technetium-99m (^{99m}Tc) pyrophosphate scanning, also known as *hot spot imaging* or *PYP scanning*, helps diagnose acute myocardial injury by showing the location and size of newly damaged myocardial tissue.

How it works

- ^{99m}Tc pyrophosphate is injected into the patient.
- Isotopes are absorbed by damaged cells.
- Damaged areas show as orange to bright red spots on the image.
- The scan reveals transmural, right ventricular, and posterior infarctions.
- Ventricular aneurysms and tumors are also visible.

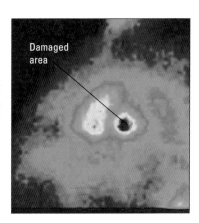

Damaged area

Test tip

Tell your patient to expect to lie on his or her back with the arms above the head during and up to 30 minutes after the test. This allows the scanner to move 360 degrees around the body.

TI^{201} + MI = COLD

Also known as *cold spot imaging,* thallium (Tl^{201}) scanning evaluates myocardial blood flow and myocardial cell status.

How it works

- Tl^{201} is injected into the patient.
- Isotopes are rapidly absorbed by healthy heart tissue and emit gamma rays. Unhealthy tissue slowly absorbs isotopes.
- Damaged areas show as **dark** spots on the image.
- The scan reveals ischemic and infarcted areas.
- The test is also used to evaluate ventricular function and the presence of pericardial effusion.

Test tip

If your patient can't raise the arms, one-dimensional Tl^{201} scanning can still be done. Pictures are taken from three different views (called *planar imaging*).

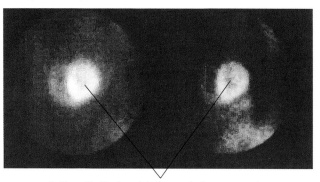

Uniform distribution of the isotope indicates normal blood flow to the left ventricle.

Chest radiography

One of the most common and cost-effective tests used to help diagnose heart disease is chest radiography. In the posterior-anterior chest X-ray view, a small dose of ionizing radiation is passed through the chest from the patient's back to the front. Structures that absorb the radiation (such as bone) appear brighter than less dense tissues (such as the lungs). Often, one or more lateral views of the chest are also included.

Purposes

- Help determine the size and shape of the heart, great vessels, and sometimes the lungs, possibly revealing signs of fluid overload or pericardial fluid
- May reveal evidence of tumors or calcifications
- Help check the placement of defibrillators, pacemakers, and invasive catheters
- Help diagnose valvular heart disease, congenital malformations, aneurysm formation, pericarditis, cardiomyopathy, heart failure, some cancers, and various lung diseases

The patient in this X-ray has situs inversus, with right-to-left reversal of all of the abdominal and thoracic contents. When the heart is found in the right chest like this, it's known as dextrocardia.

Normal chest X-ray

- Aortic arch
- Pulmonary artery
- Left atrium
- Left ventricle

X-ray showing dextrocardia

- Right sided heart
- Liver
- Stomach

Intravascular ultrasonography

In intravascular ultrasonography (IVUS), a small ultrasound transducer attached to the end of a catheter is inserted during cardiac catheterization. The catheter is commonly introduced into the femoral artery and then advanced and threaded into the coronary arteries. The transducer emits high-frequency sound waves that bounce off the arterial walls and return to the transducer, creating images of the walls from the inside out.

IVUS is often performed in conjunction with percutaneous coronary interventions such as angioplasty. It's helpful in identifying the type and amount of atherosclerosis or any other abnormalities of the arterial lumen. IVUS can also be used to evaluate stent patency and blockages following stent placement.

IVUS image of descending thoracic aorta

Intravascular ultrasound transducer

Early atheroma formation

Thoracic aorta

Wow, I'm having tunnel vision. In this image, the ultrasound transducer can be seen in the center of the smooth, circular, aortic lumen. But note the echoes in the lumen, which indicate intimal thickening and early atheroma formation.

Noninvasive Doppler ultrasonography

Duplex scan ultrasonography

Duplex scan ultrasonography involves the use of high-frequency sound waves to image and evaluate blood flow in the major arteries and veins of the abdomen, visceral organs, and extremities (arms and legs) and in the extracranial cerebrovascular system (neck). This non-invasive test uses ultrasound to create images of the vessels and deter-mine the speed, direction, and pattern of blood flow through them. Arterial duplex scans can be used to detect arterial plaque, arteriove-nous fistulas, aneurysms, and carotid body tumors. Venous duplex scans can be used to evaluate venous insufficiency and venous thrombosis.

> Measurement of systolic pressure with a Doppler transducer helps detect the presence, location, and extent of peripheral arterial occlusive disease.

A handheld transducer directs high-frequency sound waves to the artery or vein being tested.

The sound waves strike moving RBCs.

The computer then processes the sound waves to permit direct listening and graphic recording of blood flow.

The sound waves are reflected back to the transducer at frequencies that correspond to blood flow velocity through the vessel.

Pulse volume recorder testing

Pulse volume recorder testing uses a hand-held Doppler to obtain a quantitative recording of changes in blood volume or flow to an extremity.

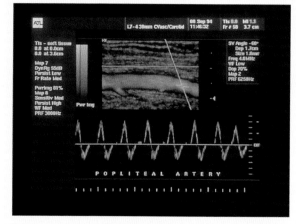

Duplex scan of popliteal artery
Color flow duplex image of popliteal artery with normal tripha-sic spectral waveform.

Measuring the ankle-brachial index

A Doppler ultrasound device can also be used to measure ankle-brachial index (ABI) to help identify peripheral vascular disease. To perform this test, follow these steps.

1 Explain the procedure to the patient.

2 Gather your materials.

3 Wash your hands.

4 Place the patient in the supine position.

5 Apply warm conductivity gel to the patient's arm where the brachial pulse has been palpated and then obtain and record the systolic reading.

6 Locate the posterior tibial pulse and repeat the procedure, recording your reading.

7 Locate the dorsalis pedis pulse and repeat the procedure.

8 Use the chart at right to calculate the ABI.

9 Document your findings.

Calculating ABI

To calculate ABI, divide the higher systolic pressure obtained for each leg (dorsalis pedia or posterior tibial) by the higher brachial systolic pressure.

Sample systolic readings (mm Hg)	Left	Right
Posterior tibial	128	96
Dorsalis pedis	130	90
Brachial	132	130
Calculations	$130 \div 132 = 0.98$	$96 \div 132 = 0.73$

What the results mean

- **Greater than 1.30:** Noncompressible (often seen in patients with diabetes or renal failure and in heavy smokers)
- **1.0–1.29:** Normal
- **0.91–0.99:** Borderline
- **0.41–0.90:** Mild to moderate peripheral artery disease (PAD)
- **0.00–0.40:** severe PAD

Venography

Also known as *ascending contrast phlebography*, venography is radiographic examination of veins in a lower extremity. During this test, a catheter is inserted into a vein (usually through the foot) and a contrast medium is injected. X-rays are then used to visualize the internal structures.

This test can cause a burning sensation in the vein when the contrast medium is injected. It also may require the use of a tourniquet for a while…ouch!

Contrast medium

Vein

Catheter

What's the problem?

This procedure isn't used for routine screening because it exposes the patient to relatively high doses of radiation and can cause such complications as phlebitis, local tissue damage and, occasionally, deep vein thrombosis. It's used in patients whose duplex ultrasound findings are unclear.

Peripheral arteriography

Peripheral arteriography, or *angiography*, is the injection of a contrast medium into the peripheral arteries accompanied by cineangiograms (rapidly changing movies on an intensified fluoroscopic screen), which record passage of the contrast medium through the vascular system. Arteriography can also be done using a magnetic resonance scanner and contrast medium.

Arteriography demonstrates the type, location, and degree of obstruction and collateral circulation. This procedure is particularly useful for monitoring chronic disease and evaluating candidates for reconstructive surgery.

Angiograph of the femoral artery and its branches

Patient's right leg

Patient's left leg

Be aware of the risks of injecting a contrast medium. Your patient may experience an allergic reaction to the dye, local tissue damage, bleeding or clotting at the puncture site, worsening renal function, or even a stroke.

a = Lateral circumflex femoral artery
b = Medial circumflex femoral artery
c = Femoral artery
d = Descending branch of the profunda femoris artery
e = Profunda femoris artery
f = Femoral artery

Matchmaker

Match the diagnostic test with its proper description.

1. BNP test _____

2. Echocardiography _____

3. Venography _____

4. Lipoprotein fractionation _____

5. MUGA scanning _____

6. aPTT _____

7. 12-lead ECG _____

A. Also known as *cardiac blood pool imaging*

B. Uses ultra-high-frequency sound waves that bounce off cardiac structures

C. Isolates and measures three types of cholesterol in blood

D. Requires using a series of electrodes to view the heart from different angles

E. Helps diagnose and grade the severity of heart failure based on hormone levels

F. Evaluates clotting factors and helps monitor response to heparin

G. Involves catheterization of a lower extremity to view veins

"X" marks the spot

Place an "X" on this illustration over the area that represents myocardial damage.

spot. See page 76.

Answers: Matchmaker 1. E, 2. B, 3. G, 4. C, 5. A, 6. F, 7. D; "X" marks the

Suggested References

Adams, J.E., III, Abendschein, D.R., & Jaffe, A.S. Biochemical Markers of Myocardial Injury. Is MB Creatine Kinase the Choice for the 1990s? *Circulation* 88(2):750–763, 1993.

http://www.healthline.com/health/electrolyte-disorders#types4

http://www.mayoclinic.org/tests-procedures/prothrombin-time/details/results/rsc-20163828

http://www.heart.org/HEARTORG/Conditions/HeartAttack/DiagnosingaHeartAttack/Transesophageal-Echocardiography TEE_UCM_441655_Article.jsp#.WYeJfF-GQyss

https://www.unitypoint.org/cedarrapids/filesimages/Physician%20and%20Clinics/Cardiology/Patient%20ed%202016/UPC_Cardiac%20Blood%20Pool_5-13.pdf

Chapter 4

ECG interpretation

Cardiac monitoring

Electrocardiography is used to diagnose and monitor cardiac disorders. When a patient is hospitalized, the first step is to begin continuous cardiac monitoring. In a hardwire system, the patient is connected directly to an electrocardiograph (ECG) by electrodes, leadwires, and a monitor cable. Most monitoring systems use three or five leads and provide a continuous readout of one or more leads simultaneously. Lead selection is based on the patient's clinical situation. Lead V_1 or V_6 and an appropriate limb lead are usually used.

> Make sure that all electrical equipment and outlets are grounded to avoid electric shock and interference.

Monitoring channel 1   Monitoring channel 2

Connections to patient

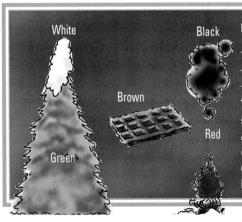

memory board

To remember where to place the electrodes in a five-electrode configuration, start by thinking of the phrase "white to the upper right." Then think of snow over trees (white electrode above green electrode) and smoke over fire (black electrode above red electrode). Of course, chocolate (brown electrode) lies in the center, close to the heart.

Leading leads

These illustrations show the heart views obtained by various monitoring leads as well as the best uses for each. Current, moving from negative to positive, makes an upward deflection of the complexes on the ECG paper; current, moving from positive to negative, makes a downward deflection on the ECG paper.

Lead I

Best for detecting atrial arrhythmias and hemiblocks

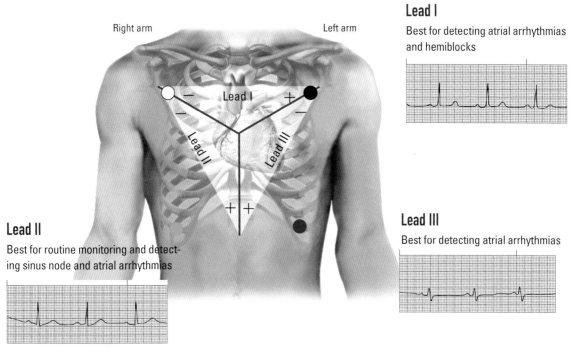

Lead II

Best for routine monitoring and detecting sinus node and atrial arrhythmias

Lead III

Best for detecting atrial arrhythmias

Viewing V_6 requires moving the chest lead from the V_1 precordial position to the V_6 precordial position.

Lead V_1

Best for detecting bundle-branch blocks, ventricular arrhythmias, and for differentiating ventricular from supraventricular tachycardia

Lead V_6

Best for ventricular conduction changes

Troubleshooting monitor problems

What you see	What might cause it	What to do about it
Artifact (waveform interference) 	• Physical activity	• Assess the patient for brushing teeth, scratching electrodes, moving around.
	• Seizures	• If the patient is having a seizure, notify the doctor and intervene as ordered.
	• Chills	• Keep the patient warm. Maintain position of cables off the chest and abdomen if possible.
	• Anxiety	• Encourage the patient to relax. Notify health care provider if needed.
	• Altered body temperature	• Assess temperature, may need different electrodes.
	• Increased or decreased	• Check the electrodes and reapply them if needed. Clean the skin well.
	• Improper electrode application	• Check the electrode gel. If the gel is dry, apply new electrodes.
	• Short circuit in leadwires or cable	• Replace broken equipment.
	• Electrical interference from other electrical equipment in the room	• Make sure all electrical equipment is attached to a common ground. • Notify the biomedical department.
False high-rate alarm	• Gain setting too high, particularly with MCL_1 setting	• Assess the patient for signs and symptoms of hyperkalemia. • Decrease gain. • Move electrodes further apart.
Weak signals	• Improper electrode application • QRS complex too small to register	• Reapply the electrodes. • Reset gain so that the height of the complex is >1 mV. • Try monitoring the patient on another lead. Move electrodes closer together.
	• Wire or cable failure	• Replace any faulty wires or cables.

What you see	What might cause it	What to do about it
Wandering baseline 	• Patient restlessness • Improper electrode application; electrode positioned over bone	• Encourage the patient to relax. • Reposition improperly placed electrodes. If system has respiratory lead, reposition.
Fuzzy baseline (electrical interference)	• Electrical interference from other equipment in the room • Improper grounding of the patient's bed • Electrode malfunction	• Ensure that all electrical equipment is attached to a common ground. • Ensure that the bed ground is attached to the room's common ground. • Replace the electrodes.
Baseline (no waveform)	• Improper electrode placement • Disconnected electrode • Dry electrode gel • Wire or cable failure	• Reposition improperly placed electrodes. • Check if electrodes are disconnected. Reapply them as necessary. • Check electrode gel. If the gel is dry, apply new electrodes. • Replace faulty wires or cables.

Note: When electrodes need to be changed, remember to change all of the leads at the same time. You never just change 1 or 2 of the leads.

Remember to treat the patient, not the monitor.

Rhythm strips

In electrocardiography, the electrical activity of the heart is displayed on a monitoring screen and can be printed onto a rhythm strip.

Worth the paper it's printed on

ECG paper consists of horizontal and vertical lines that form a grid. The top of the ECG paper has timing marks that represent 3-second intervals.

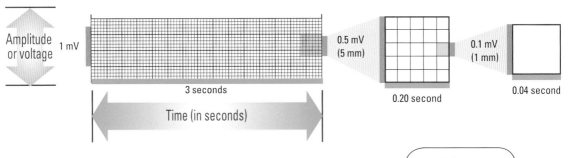

Vertical axis

The vertical axis measures amplitude in millimeters (mm) or electrical voltage in millivolts (mV). To determine the amplitude of a wave, segment, or interval, count the number of small blocks from the baseline to the highest or lowest point of the wave, segment, or interval.

Horizontal axis

The horizontal axis of the ECG strip represents time. When measuring or calculating a patient's heart rate, a 6-second strip consisting of 30 large blocks is usually used (a 3-second strip is shown above).

He's got rhythm. He's got music. Who could ask for anything more?

ECG components

8-step method

Evaluate atrial and ventricular rhythms

For the atrial rhythm, use a pair of calipers to measure the interval between P waves (P-P interval) in several ECG cycles. Set the calipers at the same point—at the beginning of the P wave or on its peak. The P wave should occur at regular intervals, with only small variations associated with respiration.

To check the ventricular rhythm, use calipers to measure the R-R intervals. Remember to place the calipers on the same point of the QRS complex. If the R-R intervals remain consistent, the ventricular rhythm is regular.

Evaluate the P wave

Observe the P wave's size, shape, and location in the waveform. If each QRS complex has a P wave, the sinoatrial (SA) node is initiating the electrical impulse, as it should be.

When using calipers to evaluate atrial rhythm, don't lift the calipers. Instead, rotate one of its legs to the next P wave to ensure accurate measurements.

Determine atrial and ventricular rates

To determine the atrial rate when the heart rate is regular, count the number of small squares between identical points on two consecutive P waves and then divide 1,500 by that number. To determine the ventricular rate, use the same method with two consecutive R waves.

Calculating rates

Three methods can be used to calculate the atrial or ventricular rate.

6-Second method
The 6-second method is useful for estimating the rate of an irregular rhythm. Count the number of P waves or R waves in two consecutive 3-second intervals, or 6-second, and then multiply by 10. The P wave calculation estimates the atrial rate, and the R wave calculation estimates the ventricular rate.

1,500 method
The 1,500 method, described above in step 2, is the most accurate method for regular rhythms, but it takes a little longer to calculate. First, count the number of small squares between two consecutive P waves, at the beginning of the P wave or on its peak, using either the apex of the wave or the initial upstroke of the wave. Then, divide 1,500 by that number to get the atrial rate. You can use the same method with two consecutive R waves to calculate the ventricular rate.

Sequence method
The sequence method is also only accurate at estimating regular rhythms. First, find a P wave that peaks on a heavy black line. Assign the following numbers to the next six heavy black lines: 300, 150, 100, 75, 60, and 50. Then, find the next P-wave peak. Estimate the rate based on the number assigned to the nearest heavy black line.

Calculate the PR interval

Count the number of small squares between the beginning of the P wave and the beginning of the QRS complex. Multiply the number of squares by 0.04 second. The normal interval is between 0.12 and 0.20 second, or between 3 and 5 small squares.

Calculate the duration of the QRS complex

Count the number of squares between the beginning and the end of the QRS complex and multiply that number by 0.04 second. A normal QRS complex is less than 0.12 second, or less than 3 small squares wide. Some references specify 0.06 to 0.10 second as the normal duration of the QRS complex. Check to see if all QRS complexes are the same size and shape, and note if a complex appears after every P wave.

Evaluate the T wave

Check that T waves are present and have a normal shape, normal amplitude, and the same deflection as QRS complexes.

Calculate the duration of the QT interval

Count the number of squares from the beginning of the QRS complex to the end of the T wave. Multiply this number by 0.04 second. The normal range is 0.36 to 0.44 second, or 9 to 11 small squares wide.

Evaluate other components

Quickly look for abnormally conducted beats and other abnormalities. Then, make sure that the waveform doesn't reflect problems with the monitor. Next, check the ST segment for abnormalities and look for a U wave. Finally, interpret the rhythm according to site of rhythm origin, rate, and rhythm.

Arrhythmias

Cardiac arrhythmias are variations in the normal pattern of electrical stimulation of the heart. Arrhythmias range from mild, causing no symptoms and requiring no treatment (such as sinus arrhythmia), to those that require emergency intervention and may cause death (such as ventricular fibrillation).

Arrhythmia locations

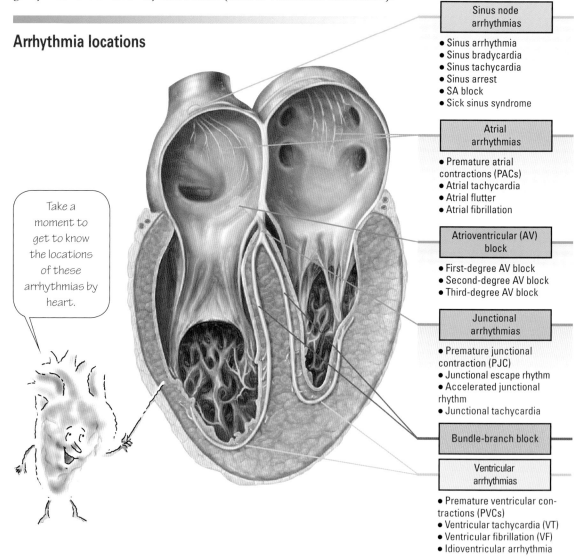

Take a moment to get to know the locations of these arrhythmias by heart.

Sinus node arrhythmias

- Sinus arrhythmia
- Sinus bradycardia
- Sinus tachycardia
- Sinus arrest
- SA block
- Sick sinus syndrome

Atrial arrhythmias

- Premature atrial contractions (PACs)
- Atrial tachycardia
- Atrial flutter
- Atrial fibrillation

Atrioventricular (AV) block

- First-degree AV block
- Second-degree AV block
- Third-degree AV block

Junctional arrhythmias

- Premature junctional contraction (PJC)
- Junctional escape rhythm
- Accelerated junctional rhythm
- Junctional tachycardia

Bundle-branch block

Ventricular arrhythmias

- Premature ventricular contractions (PVCs)
- Ventricular tachycardia (VT)
- Ventricular fibrillation (VF)
- Idioventricular arrhythmia

Sinus node arrhythmias

When the heart functions normally, the SA node, also called the *sinus node,* acts as the primary pacemaker. The SA node assumes this role because its automatic firing rate (60 to 100 beats/min in an adult at rest) exceeds that of the heart's other pacemakers. Sinus node arrhythmias occur when the node's firing rate increases or decreases.

Pacemaker rates

Pacemaker	Rate (beats/min)
SA node	60 to 100
AV node	40 to 60
Purkinje fibers	20 to 40

Sinus arrhythmia

In sinus arrhythmia, the SA node fires irregularly. When sinus arrhythmia is related to respirations, heart rate increases with inspiration and decreases with expiration, as shown at right. Sinus arrhythmia may be caused by inferior wall myocardial infarction (MI), use of digoxin (Lanoxin) or morphine (Roxanol), and increased intracranial pressure. If sinus arrhythmia is unrelated to respiration, the underlying cause may require treatment.

The cyclic irregular rhythm varies with the respiratory cycle.

Expiration   Inspiration   Expiration

Rhythm

- Irregular
- Corresponds to the respiratory cycle
- P-P interval and R-R interval shorter during respiratory inspiration; longer during expiration
- Difference between longest and shortest P-P interval exceeds 0.12 second

Rate

- Usually within normal limits (60 to 100 beats/min)
- Varies with respiration (increases during inspiration; decreases during expiration due to the effect on the vagus nerve)

P wave

- Normal size
- Normal configuration
- P wave before each QRS complex

PR interval

- May vary slightly
- Within normal limits

QRS complex

- Preceded by P wave

T wave

- Normal size
- Normal configuration

QT interval

- May vary slightly
- Usually within normal limits

Other

- Phasic slowing and quickening

Sinus bradycardia

Sinus bradycardia is a heart rate less than 60 beats/min. This may be a normal cardiac rhythm for some individuals, such as very fit athletes. If the heart rate decreases abnormally, to rates below 45 beats/min, in individuals who are not athletes, they may exhibit signs and symptoms of decreased cardiac output and hypotension, such as dizziness, confusion, and, possibly, syncope.

A normal P wave precedes each QRS complex.

The rhythm is regular, with a rate below 60 beats/min.

 ## Rhythm
- Regular

 ## Rate
- Less than 60 beats/min

 ## P wave
- Normal size
- Normal configuration
- P wave before each QRS complex

 ## PR interval
- Within normal limits
- Constant

 ## QRS complex
- Normal duration
- Normal configuration

T wave
- Normal size
- Normal configuration

 ## QT interval
- Within normal limits
- Possibly prolonged

Heart rates in children

Heart rate varies considerably with age, so evaluate bradycardia and tachycardia in context — the definitions of these in children are different than in an adult. For example, bradycardia may occur in a healthy infant during sleep; tachycardia may be a normal response when a child is crying or otherwise upset.

Age	Normal (beats/min)
Neonate	80 to 160
1 wk to 3 mo	80 to 220
3 mo to 2 yr	70 to 150
2 to 10 yr	60 to 110
>10 yr	50 to 100

Sinus tachycardia

Sinus tachycardia in an adult is characterized by a sinus rate greater than 100 beats/min. The rate rarely exceeds 180 beats/min, except during strenuous exercise.

Sinus tachycardia may be a normal response, such as with a fever. However, in a patient who has had an acute MI, it suggests massive heart damage. Persistent tachycardia may signal impending heart failure or cardiogenic shock.

A normal P wave precedes each QRS complex.

The rhythm is regular, with a rate above 100 beats/min.

 ### Rhythm
- Regular

Rate
- Greater than 100 beats/min

P wave
- Normal size
- Normal configuration
- May increase in amplitude
- Precedes each QRS complex
- As heart rate increases, possibly superimposed on preceding T wave and difficult to identify

 ### PR interval
- Within normal limits
- Constant

 ### QRS complex
- Normal duration
- Normal configuration

 ### T wave
- Normal size
- Normal configuration

 ### QT interval
- Within normal limits
- Commonly shortened

Sinus arrest

Atrial standstill occurs when the atria aren't stimulated and an entire PQRST complex is missing from an otherwise normal ECG strip. Atrial standstill is called *sinus pause* if one or two beats aren't formed and *sinus arrest* when three or more beats aren't formed. Causes of sinus arrest include hypoxia, acute infection, heart disease or MI damaging the SA node, use of some drugs, and vagal stimulation.

The rhythm is regular.   The P wave is absent.   The QRS complex is absent.

The rate is normal.

Rhythm

- Regular except during arrest (irregular as a result of missing complexes or an escape beat from the AV node or ventricle, firing as a "back up" pacemaker)

Rate

- Usually within normal limits before arrest
- Length or frequency of pause may result in bradycardia

P wave

- Absent during arrest
- When present, normal size and configuration

PR interval

- Within normal limits when a P wave is present

QRS complex

- When present, normal duration and configuration
- Absent during arrest

T wave

- When present, normal size and configuration
- Absent during arrest

QT interval

- When present, within normal limits
- Absent during arrest

Other

- Pause not a multiple of the underlying P-P intervals
- Junctional escape beats possibly occurring at the end of pause

Stop. You're under arrest!

memory board

When your patient experiences sinus arrest, use this acronym to remember the characteristics and ways to **ARREST** the situation:

Absence of three or more PQRST complexes is involved.

Rate is slowed.

Rhythm is irregular.

Excess digoxin (Lanoxin), procainamide (Pronestyl), or other antiarrhythmics may be the cause.

Syncope, dizziness, confusion, angina, or heart failure may occur.

Treat with atropine and a pacemaker if the patient is unstable.

SA block

In SA block, the SA node discharges impulses at regular intervals, but some of those impulses are delayed on the way to the atria. The most common block is the *SA exit block*. SA block may result from acute infection, an inferior wall MI and coronary artery disease (CAD) damaging the SA node, hypertensive heart disease, sinus node disease, or use of medications, such as beta-adrenergic blockers, calcium channel blockers, inotropics, or antiarrhythmics.

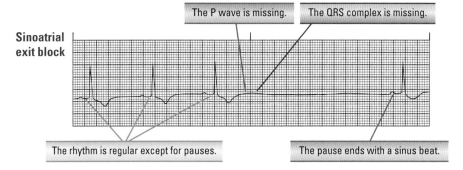

The P wave is missing. | The QRS complex is missing.

Sinoatrial exit block

The rhythm is regular except for pauses. | The pause ends with a sinus beat.

 Rhythm

- Regular except during a pause (irregular as result of a pause)

 Rate

- Usually within normal limits (60 to 100 beats/min) before a pause
- Length or frequency of pause may result in bradycardia

 P wave

- Periodically absent, with entire PQRST complex missing
- When present, normal size and configuration and precedes each QRS complex

PR interval

- Within normal limits
- Constant when a P wave is present

QRS complex

- Normal duration
- Normal configuration
- Absent during a pause

T wave

- Normal size
- Normal configuration
- Absent during a pause

QT interval

- Within normal limits
- Absent during a pause

Other

- Pause that's a multiple of the underlying P-P interval

Sinus arrest versus SA block

Sinus arrest is caused by a block in conduction, occurring high in the SA node; the impulse is blocked before it reaches the atria — so the impulse does not leave the SA node. In SA block, the impulse leaves the SA node and becomes blocked during its conduction through the atria.

Sinus arrest

SA block

Sick sinus syndrome

Also called *sinus nodal dysfunction*, sick sinus syndrome results either from a dysfunction of the sinus node's automaticity or from abnormal conduction or blockages of impulses coming out of the sinus nodal region, including one or a combination of the following conditions:

- sinus bradycardia
- SA block
- sinus arrest
- sinus bradycardia alternating with sinus tachycardia ("tachy-brady" syndrome)
- episodes of atrial tachyarrhythmias, such as atrial fibrillation and atrial flutter
- failure of the sinus node to increase the heart rate with exercise.

The rate is fast.

The P wave varies with the rhythm.

The rate is slow.

The sinus node doesn't fire, causing a sinus pause.

Rhythm

- Irregular
- Sinus pauses
- Abrupt rate changes

Rate

- Fast, slow, or alternating
- Interrupted by a long sinus pause

P wave

- Varies with rhythm changes
- May be normal size and configuration
- May be absent
- Usually precedes each QRS complex

PR interval

- Usually within normal limits
- Varies with rhythm changes

QRS complex

- Duration within normal limits
- Varies with rhythm changes
- Normal configuration

T wave

- Normal size
- Normal configuration

QT interval

- Usually within normal limits
- Varies with rhythm changes

Other

- Usually more than one arrhythmia on a 6-second strip

Recognizing an embolism

When caring for a patient with sick sinus syndrome, stay alert for signs and symptoms of an embolism, especially if the patient has atrial fibrillation. Clots that form in the heart can break off and travel through the bloodstream, blocking blood supply to the lungs, heart, brain, kidneys, intestines, and other organs.

Assess early

Assess the patient for neurologic changes (confusion, vision disturbances, weakness) and general symptoms (chest pain, dyspnea, tachypnea, tachycardia, acute onset of pain). Early recognition allows for prompt treatment.

Atrial arrhythmias

The most common cardiac rhythm disturbances, atrial arrhythmias, result from impulses originating in areas outside the SA node. They can affect ventricular filling time and diminish the strength of the atrial kick (the contraction that normally provides the ventricles with about 30% of their blood), resulting in decreased cardiac output.

Mechanisms of atrial arrhythmias

Mechanism	Characteristics	Possible causes
Altered automaticity	♥ Ability of atrial cardiac cells to initiate impulses on their own increases, triggering abnormal impulses.	♥ Hypoxia ♥ Hypocalcemia ♥ Digoxin (Lanoxin) toxicity ♥ Conditions that diminish sinoatrial node function
Reentry	♥ The impulse remains active enough to produce another impulse during myocardial repolarization. ♥ The impulse does not stop or die out, as it normally would. This creates a loop of repeated depolarizations until it is interrupted.	♥ Coronary artery disease ♥ Cardiomyopathy ♥ Myocardial infarction
Afterdepolarization	♥ An injured cell only partly repolarizes. ♥ Partial repolarization can lead to a repetitive ectopic firing called *triggered activity*. ♥ Triggered activity produces depolarization and can lead to atrial or ventricular tachycardia.	♥ Cell injury ♥ Digoxin (Lanoxin) toxicity

Premature atrial contractions (PACs)

PACs originate from an irritable spot, or *focus*, in the atria that takes over as pacemaker for one or more beats. In a patient with heart disease, PACs may lead to more serious arrhythmias, such as atrial fibrillation and atrial flutter. In a patient who has had an acute MI, PACs can serve as an early sign of heart failure or an electrolyte imbalance.

The rhythm is irregular.

Premature and abnormally shaped P waves occur.

Rhythm

- Atrial: Irregular
- Ventricular: Irregular
- Underlying: Possibly regular

Rate

- Atrial and ventricular: Vary with underlying rhythm

P wave

- Premature
- Abnormal configuration compared to a sinus P wave
- If varying configurations, multiple ectopic sites
- May be hidden in preceding T wave

PR interval

- Usually within normal limits
- May be shortened or slightly prolonged for the ectopic beat

QRS complex

- Conducted: Duration and configuration usually normal
- Nonconducted: No QRS complex follows PAC

T wave

- Usually normal
- May be distorted if P wave is hidden in T wave during a PAC

QT interval

- Usually within normal limits

Other

- May be a single beat
- May be bigeminal (every other beat premature)
- May be trigeminal (every third beat premature)
- May be quadrigeminal (every fourth beat premature)
- May occur in couplets (pairs)
- Three or more in a row: atrial tachycardia

Atrial tachycardia

Atrial tachycardia is a supraventricular tachycardia characterized by an atrial rate of 150 to 250 beats/min. Three types of atrial tachycardia exist: atrial tachycardia with block, multifocal atrial tachycardia (MAT, or *chaotic atrial tachycardia*), and paroxysmal atrial tachycardia (PAT). In atrial tachycardia with block, the number of P waves for each QRS complex may vary, depending if the block is regular. The most common block is a 2:1, with two atrial contractions for every ventricular contraction. In MAT, the shape of the P waves varies and atrial and ventricular contractions are irregular. The distinguishing characteristic of PAT is that tachycardia starts and stops suddenly in periods of normal sinus rhythm.

> The P wave may hide in the preceding T wave.

> The rate is between 150 and 250 beats/min.

 ## Rhythm

- Atrial: Usually regular
- Ventricular: Regular or irregular depending on AV conduction ratio and type of atrial tachycardia

 ## Rate

- Atrial: Three or more consecutive ectopic atrial beats at 150 to 250 beats/min; rarely exceeds 250 beats/min
- Ventricular: Varies, depending on AV conduction ratio

 ## P wave

- Deviates from normal appearance
- May be hidden in preceding T wave
- If visible, usually upright and precedes each QRS complex

PR interval

- May be difficult to measure if P wave can't be distinguished from preceding T wave

QRS complex

- Usually normal duration and configuration
- May be abnormal if impulses conducted abnormally through ventricles

 ## T wave

- Usually visible
- May be distorted by P wave
- May be inverted if ischemia is present

QT interval

- Usually within normal limits
- May be shorter because of rapid rate

 ## Other

- May be difficult to differentiate atrial tachycardia with block from sinus arrhythmia with U waves

Atrial flutter

Atrial flutter, a supraventricular tachycardia, is characterized by an atrial rate of 250 to 350 beats/min, although it's generally around 300 beats/min. The clinical significance of atrial flutter is determined by the number of impulses conducted through the node — expressed as a conduction ratio (for example, 2:1 or 4:1) — and the resulting ventricular rate. If the ventricular rate is too slow (<40 beats/min) or too fast (more than 150 beats/min), cardiac output can be seriously compromised. Usually, the faster the ventricular rate, the more dangerous the arrhythmia.

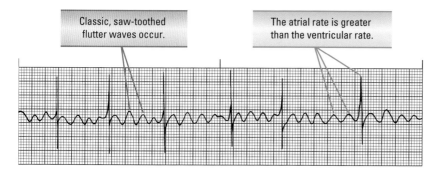

Classic, saw-toothed flutter waves occur.

The atrial rate is greater than the ventricular rate.

Rhythm

- Atrial: Regular
- Ventricular: Typically regular, although cycles may alternate (depends on AV conduction pattern)

Rate

- Atrial: 250 to 350 beats/min
- Ventricular: Usually 60 to 150 beats/min
- Usually expressed as a ratio (2:1 or 4:1, for example)

P wave

- Usually considered absent
- Saw-toothed appearance known as *flutter waves* or *F waves* are present, instead

PR interval

- Not measurable

QRS complex

- Duration: Usually within normal limits
- May be widened if flutter waves are buried within the complex

T wave

- Not identifiable

QT interval

- Not measurable because T wave not identifiable

Other

- Atrial rhythm possibly varying between a fibrillatory line and flutter waves (called *atrial fib-flutter*)

Atrial fibrillation

Sometimes called *A-fib*, atrial fibrillation is defined as chaotic, asynchronous electrical activity in the atrial tissue. This rhythm may be sustained or paroxysmal (occurring in bursts). Atrial fibrillation eliminates the atrial kick and may result in a decreased cardiac output. If the ventricular response is less than 100 beats/min, it is called *controlled atrial fibrillation*, and if greater than 100 beats/min, it is called *uncontrolled atrial fibrillation*. With an uncontrolled ventricular rate, the patient may develop heart failure, angina, or syncope. A patient with preexisting cardiac disease may develop shock and severe heart failure.

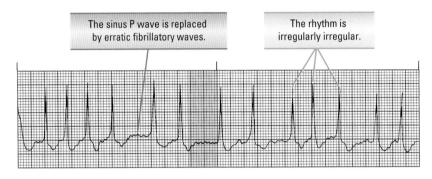

The sinus P wave is replaced by erratic fibrillatory waves.

The rhythm is irregularly irregular.

Rhythm

- Atrial: Irregularly irregular
- Ventricular: Irregularly irregular

Rate
- Atrial: Almost indiscernible, usually above 400 beats/min; far exceeds ventricular rate because most impulses aren't conducted through the atrio-ventricular junction
- Ventricular: Usually 100 to 150 beats/min but can be below 100 beats/min

P wave
- Absent
- Replaced by baseline fibrillatory waves, or F waves, that represent atrial tetanization from rapid atrial depolarizations

PR interval

- Indiscernible

QRS complex
- Duration and configuration usually normal

T wave
- Indiscernible

QT interval
- Not measurable

Other
- Atrial rhythm possibly varying between fibrillatory line and flutter waves (called atrial fib-flutter)
- May be difficult to differentiate atrial fibrillation from atrial flutter and multifocal atrial tachycardia

Untreated, A-fib may lead to cardiovascular collapse, thrombus formation, and embolism. If the patient remains in A-fib for 48 hours, anticoagulation is usually recommended.

Atrioventricular block (AV block)

AV heart block results from an interruption in the conduction of impulses between the atria and ventricles. It can be partial or total, can delay conduction, and can occur at the AV node, bundle of His, or bundle branches. When impulses from the SA node are blocked at the AV node or below, atrial rates are commonly normal (60 to 100 beats/min). The clinical effects of the block depend on how many impulses are completely blocked, how slow the resulting ventricular rate is, and how the block ultimately affects the heart function. A slow ventricular rate can decrease cardiac output, possibly causing light-headedness, hypotension, and confusion.

The severity, or degree, of an AV block is measured according to how well the node conducts impulses.

Comparing degrees of AV block

Type	Distinguishing characteristic	Possible causes
First	♥ PR interval >0.20 second Considered a "delay" rather than a block	♥ Degenerative changes ♥ Drugs: beta-adrenergic blockers, calcium channel blockers, digoxin ♥ MI ♥ Myocarditis
Type I second degree	♥ Progressive prolongation of PR interval until P wave occurs without a QRS complex (dropped beat)	♥ CAD ♥ Drugs: beta-adrenergic blockers, calcium channel blockers, digoxin ♥ Increased parasympathetic tone ♥ Inferior wall MI ♥ Rheumatic fever
Type II second degree	♥ Constant PR interval for conducted beats ♥ Periodic nonconducted P wave (dropped beat)	♥ Anterior wall MI (LAD artery) ♥ Degenerative changes in conduction system ♥ Organic heart disease ♥ Severe CAD
Third degree	♥ No relationship between P wave and QRS complex ♥ Independent beating of atria and ventricles	**At AV node level** ♥ AV node damage ♥ Increased parasympathetic tone ♥ Inferior wall MI ♥ Drug toxicity **At infranodal level** ♥ Extensive anterior wall MI

First-degree AV block

First-degree AV block occurs when impulses from the atria are consistently delayed during conduction through the AV node. The least dangerous type of AV block, first-degree AV block, can progress to a more severe block.

The PR interval is greater than 0.20 second.

The rhythm is regular.

Rhythm

- Regular

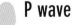
Rate

- Within normal limits
- Atrial the same as ventricular

P wave

- Normal size
- Normal configuration
- Each followed by a QRS complex

PR interval

- Prolonged
- More than 0.20 second
- Constant

QRS complex

- Within normal limits (0.08 to 0.10 second) if conduction delay occurs in AV node
- If more than 0.12 second, conduction delay may be in His-Purkinje system

T wave

- Normal size
- Normal configuration
- May be abnormal if QRS complex is prolonged

QT interval

- Within normal limits

Type I second-degree AV block

Also called *Wenckebach* or *Mobitz type I block*, type I second-degree AV block occurs when each successive impulse from the SA node is delayed slightly longer than the previous impulse. That pattern continues until an impulse fails to be conducted to the ventricles, the QRS complex is "dropped," and the cycle then repeats.

The PR interval gets progressively longer...

...until a QRS complex is dropped.

Rhythm

- Atrial: Regular
- Ventricular: Irregular

Rate

- Atrial rate exceeds ventricular rate because of nonconducted beats
- Both rates usually within normal limits

P wave

- Normal size
- Normal configuration
- Each followed by a QRS complex, except when the P wave is blocked and the QRS drops

PR interval

- Progressively longer with each cycle until a P wave appears without a QRS complex
- Commonly described as "long, longer, dropped"
- Slight variation in delay from cycle to cycle
- After the nonconducted beat, shorter than the interval preceding it

QRS complex

- Within normal limits
- Periodically absent when dropped from the rhythm.

T wave

- Normal size
- Normal configuration
- Deflection may be opposite that of the QRS complex

QT interval

- Usually within normal limits

Other

- Wenckebach pattern of grouped beats (footprints of Wenckebach)
- Progressive shortening of R-R interval until a QRS complex is dropped; cycle then repeats

Type I second-degree AV block may occur normally in an otherwise healthy person.

Type II second-degree AV block

Type II second-degree AV block, also known as *Mobitz type II block*, is less common than type I but is more serious. The ventricular rate is usually slower than in type I. Cardiac output is diminished, which may cause the patient to become symptomatic, and it may progress to a more serious form of block.

The atrial rhythm is regular...

...but the ventricular rhythm is irregular.

The PR interval is constant.

A QRS complex should be here.

Rhythm

- Atrial: Regular
- Ventricular: Irregular
- Pauses correspond to dropped beat
- Irregular when block is intermittent or conduction ratio is variable
- Regular when conduction ratio, or block, is consistent, such as 2:1 or 3:1

Rate

- Atrial exceeds ventricular
- Both may be within normal limits

P wave

- Normal size
- Normal configuration
- Some not followed by a QRS complex

PR interval

- Usually within normal limits but may be prolonged
- Constant for conducted beats
- May be shortened after a nonconducted beat

QRS complex

- Within normal limits or narrow if block occurs at the bundle of His
- Widened and similar to bundle-branch block if block occurs at bundle branches
- Periodically absent

T wave

- Normal size
- Normal configuration

QT interval

- Within normal limits

Other

- No variation in PR and R-R intervals before a dropped beat, so no warning occurs
- R-R interval that contains nonconducted P wave equaling two normal R-R intervals

Third-degree AV block

Also called *complete heart block*, third-degree AV block occurs when impulses from the atria are completely blocked at the AV node and are not conducted to the ventricles. The ventricular rhythm may originate from the AV node or the Purkinje system. Patients with very slow ventricular rates may have a diminished cardiac output, causing symptoms such as light-headedness, poor exercise tolerance, and shortness of breath in patients. More serious symptoms, including syncope, chest pain, and hypotension, are also common.

The atrial rhythm is regular.

The P wave occurs without a QRS complex.

The ventricular rhythm is regular.

Rhythm

- Atrial: Regular
- Ventricular: Regular

Rate

- Atrial: 60 to 100 beats/min (atria act independently under control of sinoatrial node)
- Ventricular: Usually 40 to 60 beats/min if level is an infranodal block (a junctional escape rhythm)
- Ventricular: Usually less than 40 beats/min in an infranodal block, it is at the level of the bundle branches (a ventricular escape rhythm)

P wave

- Normal size
- Normal configuration
- May be buried in QRS complex or T wave

PR interval

- Not measurable

QRS complex

- Configuration depending on location of escape mechanism and origin of ventricular depolarization
- Appears normal if the block is at the level of atrioventricular node or bundle of His
- Widened if the block is at the level of the bundle branches

T wave

- Normal size
- Normal configuration
- May be abnormal if QRS complex originates in ventricle

QT interval

- Within normal limits

Other

- Atria and ventricles depolarizing from different pacemaker sites and beating independently of each other
- P waves occurring without QRS complexes

Junctional arrhythmias

Junctional arrhythmias originate in the AV junction — the area around the AV node and the bundle of His. These arrhythmias occur when the SA node fails to conduct impulses or when a block in conduction occurs. Electrical impulses may then be initiated by pacemaker cells in the AV junction in the middle of the heart. Impulses generated in this area cause the heart to depolarize abnormally. The impulse moves upward and causes backward, or retrograde, depolarization of the atria and may result in inverted (rather than upright) P waves in leads II, III, and aV$_F$. The ventricles respond normally to the stimulus, resulting in a QRS complex that usually appears normal on the rhythm strip.

Hey wait! I thought retro was in!

P-wave positions

The position of the P wave depends on whether the impulse reaches the atria or ventricles first.

Atria first

Inverted P wave before QRS complex

Simultaneous

Inverted P wave after QRS complex

Ventricles first

Inverted P wave hidden in QRS

Premature junctional contractions (PJCs)

A PJC is an ectopic beat that occurs when an irritable location within the AV junction acts as a pacemaker and fires either prematurely or out of sequence. It occurs before a normal sinus beat and causes an irregular rhythm. Although the junctional beat itself isn't recorded on the ECG strip, its effects on the timing of atrial (retrograde) and ventricular (anterograde) depolarization are seen.

> The rhythm is irregular.

> The P wave is inverted, with PR interval less than 0.12 second.

Rhythm

- Atrial: Irregular during PJCs
- Ventricular: Irregular during PJCs
- Underlying rhythm possibly regular

Rate

- Atrial: Reflects underlying rhythm
- Ventricular: Reflects underlying rhythm

P wave

- Usually inverted (leads II, III, and aV$_F$)
- May occur before, during (would be hidden in the QRS), or after QRS complex, depending on initial direction of depolarization

PR interval

- Shortened (<0.12 second) if P wave precedes QRS complex, but not a "true" PR interval, since the atrial activity did not *cause* the QRS. It is retrograde conduction
- Not measurable if no P wave precedes QRS complex

QRS complex

- Usually normal configuration and duration because ventricles usually depolarize normally

T wave

- Usually normal configuration

QT interval

- Usually within normal limits

Other

- Commonly accompanied by a compensatory pause, reflecting retrograde atrial conduction

Junctional escape rhythm

A junctional escape rhythm is a string of beats that occurs after a conduction delay from the atria. It can be caused by any condition that disturbs SA node function or enhances AV junction automaticity. A patient with a junctional escape rhythm has a slow, regular pulse rate of 40 to 60 beats/min and may be asymptomatic.

The P wave is inverted.

The rhythm is regular, with a rate of 40 to 60 beats/min.

Rhythm

- Atrial: Regular, if P waves are seen; however, they do not *cause* the QRS in this rhythm
- Ventricular: Regular

Rate

- Atrial: 40 to 60 beats/min
- Ventricular: 40 to 60 beats/min

P wave

- Usually inverted (leads II, III, and aVF), representing retrograde depolarization
- May occur before, during (would be hidden in the QRS), or after QRS complex

PR interval

- Shortened (<0.12 second) if P wave precedes QRS complex, but not a "true" PR interval, since the atrial activity did not cause the QRS. It is retrograde conduction
- Not measurable if no P wave precedes QRS complex

QRS complex

- Duration: Usually within normal limits
- Configuration: Usually normal

T wave

- Configuration: Usually normal

A close look at WPW syndrome

In Wolff-Parkinson-White (WPW) syndrome, the conducted impulse travels to the atria or ventricles via a bypass known as *Kent's bundle*. Because impulses aren't delayed at the AV node, conduction is abnormally fast. Retrograde conduction, reentry, and reentrant tachycardia can result. This syndrome is typically a congenital rhythm disorder that occurs mainly in young children and in adults ages 20 to 35.

On the ECG
- Delta wave (hallmark sign)
- Short PR interval (<0.10 second)
- Wide QRS complex (>0.10 second)

QT interval

- Usually within normal limits

Other

- Important to differentiate junctional rhythm from idioventricular rhythm (a life-threatening arrhythmia). It is usually based on the rate and QRS shape and measurement

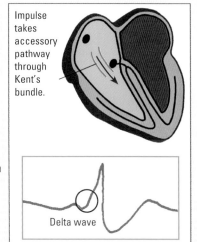

Impulse takes accessory pathway through Kent's bundle.

Delta wave

Accelerated junctional rhythm

An accelerated junctional rhythm results when an irritable focus in the AV junction speeds up and takes over as the heart's pacemaker. The atria depolarize by retrograde conduction, and the ventricles depolarize normally. The accelerated rate is usually 60 to 100 beats/min.

No P wave appears before the QRS complex.

The rhythm is regular, with a rate between 60 and 100 beats/min.

Rhythm

- Atrial: Regular
- Ventricular: Regular

Rate

- Atrial: 60 to 100 beats/min
- Ventricular: 60 to 100 beats/min

P wave

- If present, inverted in leads II, III, and aVF
- May occur before, during (would be hidden in the QRS), or after QRS complex

PR interval

- Shortened (<0.12 second) if P wave precedes QRS complex, but not a "true" PR interval, since the atrial activity did not cause the QRS. It is retrograde conduction
- Not measurable if no P wave precedes QRS complex

QRS complex

- Duration: Usually within normal limits
- Configuration: Usually normal

T wave

- Usually within normal limits

QT interval

- Usually within normal limits

Other

- Necessary to differentiate accelerated junctional rhythm from accelerated idioventricular rhythm (a possibly life-threatening arrhythmia). It is usually done by the QRS shape and measurement

The patient with accelerated junctional rhythm may be asymptomatic because the rhythm has the same rate as sinus rhythm.

Junctional tachycardia

In junctional tachycardia, three or more PJCs occur in a row. This supraventricular tachycardia occurs when an irritable focus from the AV junction overrides the SA node's ability to function as the heart's pacemaker. The atria depolarize by retrograde conduction; however, conduction through the ventricles remains normal.

The rhythm is regular, with a rate of 100 to 200 beats/min.

The P wave is inverted.

Rhythm

- Atrial: Usually regular but may be difficult to determine if P wave is hidden in QRS complex or preceding T wave
- Ventricular: Usually regular

Rate

- Atrial: Exceeds 100 beats/min (usually 100 to 200 beats/min) but may be difficult to determine if P wave isn't visible
- Ventricular: Exceeds 100 beats/min (usually 100 to 200 beats/min)

P wave

- Usually inverted in leads II, III, and aV$_F$
- May occur before, during (would be hidden in the QRS), or after QRS complex

PR interval

- Shortened (0.12 second) if P wave precedes QRS complex, but not a "true" PR interval, since the atrial activity did not *cause* the QRS. It is retrograde conduction
- Not measurable if no P wave precedes QRS complex

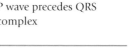
QRS complex

- Duration: Within normal limits
- Configuration: Usually normal

T wave

- Configuration: Usually normal
- May be abnormal if P wave is hidden in T wave
- May be indiscernible because of fast rate

QT interval

- Usually within normal limits

Other

- Onset possibly gradual (nonparoxysmal) or sudden (paroxysmal)

Bundle-branch block

In bundle-branch block (BBB), an impulse originates supraventricularly, and the left or the right bundle branch fails to conduct impulses. The impulse travels down the unaffected bundle branch, and then from one myocardial cell to the next, to depolarize the ventricle. Because this cell-to-cell conduction progresses much slower than the conduction along the specialized cells of the conduction system, ventricular depolarization is prolonged. A BBB that occurs low in the left bundle is called a *hemiblock* or *fascicular block*.

Right bundle-branch block

Right bundle-branch block (RBBB) may occur in patients with CAD, pulmonary embolism, or recent anterior wall MI. However, it can also occur without the presence of cardiac disease.

Left bundle-branch block

Left bundle-branch block (LBBB) never occurs normally. This block is usually caused by hypertensive heart disease, aortic stenosis, degenerative changes of the conduction system, or CAD.

Recognizing RBBB and LBBB

The normal width of a QRS complex is 0.06 to 0.10 second. However, prolonged ventricular depolarization widens the QRS complex. If the width increases to greater than 0.12 second, a bundle-branch block may be present.

In order to identify a BBB, examine lead V_1, which lies to the right of the heart, and lead V_6, which lies to the left of the heart. These leads determine whether the block is a right bundle-branch block (RBBB) or a left bundle-branch block (LBBB).

RBBB

In RBBB, V_1 shows a small r wave (showing left ventricular depolarization), followed by a small S wave, and then a large R' wave (confirming right ventricular depolarization)—rSR'. V_6 shows a widened S wave and an upright T wave.

LBBB

In LBBB, V_1 usually shows no R wave and a wide, large Q wave and may or may not have an S wave. V_6 shows slurred R waves and inverted T waves.

Ventricular arrhythmias

Ventricular arrhythmias originate in the ventricles below the bundle of His. They occur when electrical impulses depolarize the myocardium using an abnormal pathway. When electrical impulses originate in the ventricles instead of the atria, atrial kick is lost and cardiac output decreases by as much as 30%. As a result, patients may show signs and symptoms of cardiac decompensation, including hypotension, syncope, respiratory distress, and angina.

Ventricular arrhythmias are potentially deadly because the ventricles are ultimately responsible for cardiac output. Rapid recognition and treatment of ventricular arrhythmias increase the chance for successful resuscitation.

Signs and symptoms of cardiac decompensation

Hypotension and syncope   **Respiratory distress**   **Angina**

Premature ventricular contractions (PVCs)

A PVC is an ectopic beat that originates low in the ventricles and occurs earlier than normal. PVCs can occur singly, in clusters of two or more, or in repeating patterns, such as bigeminy (every other beat) or trigeminy (every third beat). PVCs that look alike originate from the same ectopic focus and are called *unifocal*. PVCs that don't look alike originate from different ectopic foci and are called *multifocal*. These beats may appear in patterns that can progress to more lethal arrhythmias.

Premature QRS complex appears wide and bizarre.

The rhythm is irregular.

Rhythm

- Atrial: Irregular during PVCs
- Ventricular: Irregular during PVCs
- Underlying rhythm may be regular

Rate

- Atrial: Reflects underlying rhythm
- Ventricular: Reflects underlying rhythm

P wave

- Usually absent in ectopic beat
- May appear after QRS complex with retrograde conduction to atria
- Usually normal if present in underlying rhythm

PR interval

- Not measurable except in underlying rhythm

QRS complex

- Occurs earlier than expected
- Duration: Exceeds 0.12 second
- Configuration: Bizarre, wide, and often oppositely deflected from the underlying QRS complex, but usually normal in underlying rhythm

T wave

- Opposite direction to QRS complex
- May trigger more serious rhythm disturbances when PVC occurs on the downslope of the preceding normal T wave (R-on-T phenomenon)

QT interval

- Not usually measured except in underlying rhythm

Other

- PVC possibly followed by full or incomplete or noncompensatory pause
- Interpolated PVC: Occurs between two normally conducted QRS complexes without great disturbance to underlying rhythm — the R-R measurement is the same
- Interpolated PVCs do not have full compensatory pauses

A compensatory pause is the interval between two normal sinus beats containing a PVC; it equals two normal sinus intervals.

Patterns of potentially dangerous PVCs

Some PVCs are more dangerous than others. Here are some potentially dangerous ones.

PVCs in a Row

Two PVCs occurring consecutively, called *paired PVCs* or a *ventricular couplet*, can produce VT because the second contraction usually meets refractory tissue. A burst, or *salvo*, of three or more PVCs in a row is considered a run of VT.

Multifocal PVCs

Multifocal PVCs arise either from different sites or from the same site via abnormal conduction and look different from one another. Multifocal PVCs may indicate acid-base disturbances, electrolyte imbalances, hypoxia, severe heart disease, or digoxin toxicity.

Bigeminy and trigeminy

PVCs that occur every other beat (bigeminy) or every third beat (trigeminy) can result in VT or VF.

R-on-T phenomenon

In R-on-T phenomenon, a PVC occurs so early that it falls on the T wave of the preceding beat. Because the cells haven't fully repolarized, VT or VF can result.

Take this info to heart

♥ Until effective treatment begins, patients with PVCs accompanied by serious symptoms should have continuous ECG monitoring and minimize activity in order to decrease oxygen demand.

♥ If the patient is discharged from the hospital on antiarrhythmic medications, patient and family member education should include follow-up appointments and lab tests, knowing when and how to activate the emergency medical system and how to perform cardiopulmonary resuscitation (CPR).

Ventricular tachycardia (VT)

In VT, commonly called *V-tach*, three or more PVCs occur in a row. This arrhythmia often precedes ventricular fibrillation and sudden cardiac death, especially in patients who are not hospitalized. It can occur in short, paroxysmal bursts lasting fewer than 30 seconds and causing few or no symptoms. Alternatively, it can be sustained, requiring immediate treatment to prevent death.

The QRS complex is wide and bizarre.

The ventricular rate is 100 to 250 beats/min.

Rhythm

- Atrial: Can't be determined
- Ventricular: Usually regular but may be slightly irregular

Rate

- Atrial: Can't be determined
- Ventricular: Usually rapid (100 to 250 beats/min)

P wave

- Usually not visible.
- If visible, not associated with QRS complex

PR interval

- Not measurable

QRS complex

- Duration: Exceeds 0.12 second
- Configuration: Usually bizarre, with increased amplitude, compared to the underlying rhythm
- Uniform in monomorphic ventricular tachycardia
- Constantly changes shape in polymorphic ventricular tachycardia

T wave

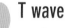

- If visible, occurs opposite the QRS complex

QT interval

- Not measurable

Other

- Ventricular flutter: A variation of VT in which a single ventricular focus fires at a rapid rate of 250 to 350 beats/min, producing a continuous, uniform waveform

Torsades de pointes

Torsades de pointes, which means "twisting of the points," is a variation of polymorphic VT that may deteriorate into VF. The cause is usually reversible — most commonly, a low serum magnesium level and use of drugs that lengthen the QT interval, such as quinidine, procainamide (Pronestyl), and sotalol (Betapace). Myocardial ischemia can also cause this arrhythmia.

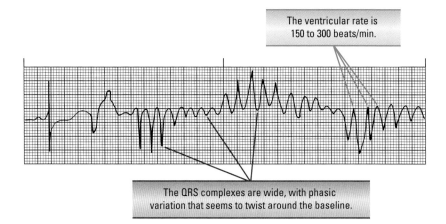

The ventricular rate is 150 to 300 beats/min.

The QRS complexes are wide, with phasic variation that seems to twist around the baseline.

Rhythm

- Atrial: Can't be determined
- Ventricular: May be regular or irregular

Rate

- Atrial: Can't be determined
- Ventricular: 150 to 300 beats/min

P wave

- Not identifiable

PR interval

- Not measurable

QRS complex

- Usually wide
- Usually a phasic variation in electrical polarity, with complexes that point downward for several beats and then upward for several beats — the "twisting" pattern

T wave

- Not discernible

QT interval

- Prolonged

Other

- May be paroxysmal, starting and stopping suddenly

Ventricular fibrillation (VF)

VF, commonly called *V-fib*, is a chaotic pattern of electrical activity in the ventricles, in which electrical impulses arise from many different foci. The ventricles quiver instead of contracting, so cardiac output falls to zero. If fibrillation continues, it leads to ventricular standstill (asystole) and death.

The presence of large fibrillatory waves indicates coarse ventricular fibrillation.

Coarse

Fine

The presence of small fibrillatory waves indicates fine ventricular fibrillation.

 ## Rhythm

- Atrial: Can't be determined
- Ventricular: No pattern or regularity, just fibrillatory waves

 ## Rate

- Atrial: Can't be determined
- Ventricular: Can't be determined

 ## P wave

- Can't be determined

 ## PR interval

- Can't be determined

QRS complex

- Can't be determined

T wave

- Can't be determined

QT interval

- Not measurable

 ## Other

- Electrical defibrillation more successful with coarse fibrillatory waves than with fine waves

If my ventricles quiver rather than contract, it's time for you to act!

Idioventricular rhythm

Called the *rhythm of last resort*, idioventricular rhythm occurs when no impulses are conducted to the ventricles from above the bundle of His and is the last rhythm before ventricular standstill, or asystole. The cells of the His-Purkinje system take over as the heart's pacemaker to generate electrical impulses.

The rate is below 40 beats/min.

The QRS complex is wide and bizarre.

 ### Rhythm
- Atrial: Usually can't be determined
- Ventricular: Usually regular

 ### Rate
- Atrial: Usually can't be determined
- Ventricular: 20 to 40 beats/min

P wave
- Usually absent

 ### PR interval
- Not measurable because of absent P wave

 ### QRS complex
- Duration: Exceeds 0.12 second because of abnormal ventricular depolarization
- Configuration: Wide and bizarre

 ### T wave
- Abnormal
- Usually deflects in opposite direction from QRS complex

 ### QT interval
- Usually prolonged

Other
- Commonly occurring with third-degree atrioventricular block
- If any P waves present, not associated with QRS complex

Asystole

Asystole is ventricular standstill. There is no electrical activity in the heart, so the patient is completely unresponsive. There is no cardiac output and no respirations.

The absence of electrical activity in the ventricles results in a nearly flat line.

Rhythm

- Atrial: Usually indiscernible
- Ventricular: Not present

Rate

- Atrial: Usually indiscernible
- Ventricular: Not present

P wave

- Usually indiscernible

PR interval

- Not measurable

QRS complex

- Absent or occasional escape beats

T wave

- Absent

QT interval

- Not measurable

Other

- Looks like a nearly flat line on a rhythm strip except with chest compressions during cardiopulmonary resuscitation
- If the patient has a pacemaker, pacer spikes may show on the strip, but no P wave or QRS complex occurs in response

Asystole should be confirmed in two different monitoring leads

When my electricity goes out, asystole results.

Color my world

Color each circle with the appropriate lead color that should be used for continuous cardiac monitoring.

Match maker

Match each of the arrhythmias shown with their correct name.

1. ____

2. ____

3. ____

____ **A.** VF

____ **B.** Atrial fibrillation

____ **C.** VT

Suggested References

Ahlert, B.J. *ECG's Made Easy*, 5th ed. St. Louis: Elsevier, 2013.

Lough, M.E., & Thompson, C. Cardiovascular diagnostic procedures. In L.D. Urden, K.M. Stacy, & M.E. Lough, eds. *Critical Care Nursing: Diagnosis and Management*. St. Louis: Elsevier, 2014:274–315.

Moseley, M.J. Dysrhythmia interpretation and management. In M.L. Sole, D.G. Klein, & M.J. Moseley, *Introduction to Critical Care Nursing*. St. Louis: Elsevier, 2017:89–129.

Sole, M.L., Klein, D.G., & Moseley, M.J. *Introduction to Critical Care Nursing*, 7th ed. St. Louis: Elsevier, 2017.

Urden, L.D., Stacy, K.M., & Lough, M.E. *Critical Care Nursing: Diagnosis and Management*. St. Louis: Elsevier, 2014.

Chapter 5

Hemodynamic monitoring

Arterial blood pressure monitoring

Hemodynamic monitoring is used to assess cardiac function and to determine the effectiveness of therapy. In arterial blood pressure monitoring, a doctor inserts a catheter into the patient's radial or femoral artery to measure systolic, diastolic, and mean pressures or to obtain samples for ABG studies. A transducer transforms the flow of blood during systole and diastole into a waveform, which appears on a monitor screen.

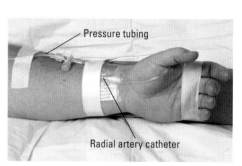

Pressure tubing

Radial artery catheter

Normal arterial pressure parameters

In general, arterial **systolic pressure** reflects the peak pressure generated by the left ventricle. It also indicates compliance of the large arteries, or the *peripheral resistance*.

Arterial **diastolic pressure** reflects the runoff velocity and elasticity of the arterial system, particularly the arterioles.

Mean arterial pressure (MAP) is the average pressure in the arterial system during systole and diastole. It reflects the driving, or *perfusion*, pressure and is determined by arterial blood volume and blood vessel elasticity and resistance.

$$MAP = \frac{\text{systolic pressure} + 2\,(\text{diastolic pressure})}{3}$$

Arterial waveform configuration

Normal arterial blood pressure produces a characteristic wave-form, representing ventricular systole and diastole. The wave-form has five distinct components, as shown below.

> Knowing the components of an arterial waveform keeps you ahead of the game on arterial pressure monitoring.

Normal arterial waveform

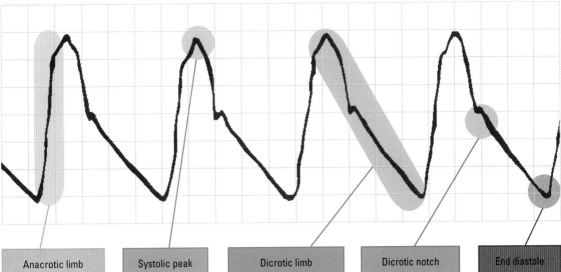

Anacrotic limb	Systolic peak	Dicrotic limb	Dicrotic notch	End diastole
The *anacrotic limb* marks the waveform's initial upstroke, which occurs as blood is rapidly ejected from the ventricle through the open aortic valve into the aorta.	Arterial pressure then rises sharply, resulting in the *systolic peak* — the waveform's highest point.	As blood continues into the peripheral vessels, arterial pressure falls and the waveform begins a downward trend, called the *dicrotic limb*. Arterial pressure usually keeps falling until pressure in the ventricle is less than pressure in the aortic root.	When ventricular pressure is lower than aortic root pressure, the aortic valve closes. This event appears as a small notch on the waveform's downside, called the *dicrotic notch*.	When the aortic valve closes, diastole begins, progressing until aortic root pressure gradually falls to its lowest point. On the waveform, this is known as *end diastole*.

Recognizing abnormal waveforms

Understanding a normal arterial waveform is relatively straightforward. Unfortunately, an abnormal waveform isn't so easy to decipher. Abnormal patterns and markings, however, may provide important diagnostic clues to the patient's cardiovascular status, or they may simply signal trouble in the monitor. Use this chart to help you recognize waveform abnormalities. *Always check the patient when an abnormal waveform is noted.*

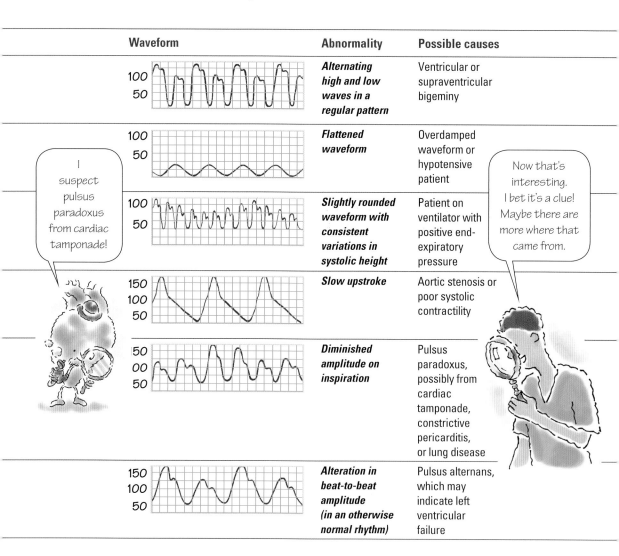

Waveform	Abnormality	Possible causes
100 50	*Alternating high and low waves in a regular pattern*	Ventricular or supraventricular bigeminy
100 50	*Flattened waveform*	Overdamped waveform or hypotensive patient
100 50	*Slightly rounded waveform with consistent variations in systolic height*	Patient on ventilator with positive end-expiratory pressure
150 100 50	*Slow upstroke*	Aortic stenosis or poor systolic contractility
50 00 50	*Diminished amplitude on inspiration*	Pulsus paradoxus, possibly from cardiac tamponade, constrictive pericarditis, or lung disease
150 100 50	*Alteration in beat-to-beat amplitude (in an otherwise normal rhythm)*	Pulsus alternans, which may indicate left ventricular failure

Pulmonary artery pressure monitoring

Continuous pulmonary artery pressure (PAP) and intermittent pulmonary artery occlusion pressure (PAOP) measurements provide important information about left ventricular function and preload.

Come equipped

PA catheter

As shown here, a pulmonary artery (PA) catheter contains several lumens. Each lumen has its own purpose (indicated in parentheses).

Balloon inflation port

Thermistor port (cardiac output)

Proximal port (PAP, CVP)

Distal port (PAP, PAOP)

Extra port (fluids, medications)

Normal PAP values

Right atrial pressure	1 to 6 mm Hg
Systolic right ventricular pressure	20 to 30 mm Hg
End-diastolic right ventricular pressure	Less than 5 mm Hg
Systolic PAP	20 to 30 mm Hg
Diastolic PAP	10 to 15 mm Hg
Mean PAP	Less than 20 mm Hg
PAOP	6 to 12 mm Hg

Normal pulmonary artery waveforms

After insertion into a large vein (usually the subclavian, jugular, or femoral vein), a PA catheter is advanced through the vena cava into the right atrium, through the right ventricle, and into a branch of the pulmonary artery. As the catheter advances through the heart chambers during insertion, the monitor shows various waveforms, described below.

When the catheter tip enters the right atrium, this waveform appears on the monitor, representing right atrial pressure.

The catheter tip enters the right atrium.

Watch the patient's ECG monitor closely. Ventricular arrhythmias can occur as the catheter passes through the right ventricle.

Next, the catheter tip reaches the right ventricle.

As the catheter tip reaches the right ventricle, you'll see a waveform with sharp systolic upstrokes and lower diastolic dips.

3

As the catheter reaches the pulmonary artery, the upstroke of the waveform becomes smoother than that of the right ventricular waveform.

The catheter floats into the pulmonary artery.

The dicrotic notch indicates closure of the pulmonic valve.

4

The catheter's balloon floats into a distal branch of the pulmonary artery. The balloon occludes the vessel because it is too narrow for it to pass.

The monitor now shows a PAOP waveform with two small uprises. The balloon is then passively deflated by simply removing the syringe, and the catheter is left in the pulmonary artery.

Identifying hemodynamic pressure monitoring problems

Problem	What might cause it	What to do about it
Line fails to flush	• Inadequate pressure from pressure bag	• Make sure the pressure bag gauge reads 300 mm Hg.
	• Blood clot in catheter	• Try to aspirate the clot with a syringe. If the line still won't flush, notify the doctor and prepare to replace the line. ***Never use a syringe to flush a hemodynamic line.***
Damped waveform	• Air bubbles	• Secure all connections. • Remove air from the lines and the transducer. • Check for and replace cracked equipment.
	• Blood flashback in line	• Make sure stopcock positions are correct; tighten loose connections and replace cracked equipment, if necessary. • Flush the line with the fast-flush valve/pig tail. • Replace the transducer if blood backs up into it.
	• Incorrect transducer position	• Make sure the transducer is kept at the level of the right atrium at all times. Improper levels give false-high or false-low pressure readings. • Reposition the catheter if it's against the vessel wall.
	• Malpositioned arterial catheter (out of blood vessel or pressed against vessel wall)	• Try to aspirate blood to confirm proper placement in the vessel. If you can't aspirate blood, notify the doctor and prepare to replace the line. ***Note: Bloody drainage at the insertion site may indicate catheter displacement. Notify the doctor immediately.***
	• Incorrect pressure scale setting	• Ensure that the scale is set for the appropriate pressure.
PAOP tracing unobtainable	• Ruptured balloon	• If you feel no resistance when injecting air or if you see blood leaking from the balloon inflation lumen, stop injecting air and notify the doctor. If the catheter is left in, label the inflation lumen with a warning not to inflate.
	• Incorrect amount of air in balloon	• Passively deflate the balloon by simply removing the syringe. Check the label on the catheter for correct volume. Reinflate slowly with the correct amount. To avoid rupturing the balloon, always utilize a PA-designated syringe.
	• Malpositioned catheter	• Notify the doctor. • Obtain a chest X-ray.
No waveform	• Defective equipment	• Check all connections. • Replace the monitor cable. • Replace the transducer.
	• Incorrectly positioned stopcock	• Ensure that the stopcock is open to the patient.
	• Clot or kink in catheter	• Check the line setup for kinks in the tubing. If none are noted, slowly aspirate for blood return. If none is noted, notify the physician.

Cardiac output monitoring

Measuring cardiac output (CO) — the amount of blood (in liters) ejected by the heart in 1 minute — helps evaluate cardiac function. Common methods for monitoring CO are the bolus thermodilution method, continuous cardiac output (CCO) monitoring PA catheter, and arterial pressure–based CO (APCO) monitoring.

> Repeat the injection procedure at least three times to obtain a mean CO value.

Bolus thermodilution method

In the bolus thermodilution method, a solution colder than the patient's blood is injected into the right atrium through a port on a pulmonary artery catheter. The catheter detects changes in temperature as the blood flows, and a computer uses this data to calculate cardiac output.

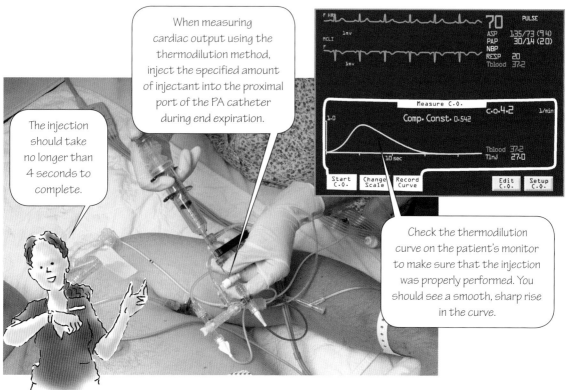

> When measuring cardiac output using the thermodilution method, inject the specified amount of injectant into the proximal port of the PA catheter during end expiration.

> The injection should take no longer than 4 seconds to complete.

> Check the thermodilution curve on the patient's monitor to make sure that the injection was properly performed. You should see a smooth, sharp rise in the curve.

A closer look at the thermodilution method

Performed at the bedside, the thermodilution method is the most practical way of evaluating the cardiac status of critically ill patients and those suspected of having cardiac disease. This illustration shows the path of the injectate solution through the heart during thermodilution CO monitoring.

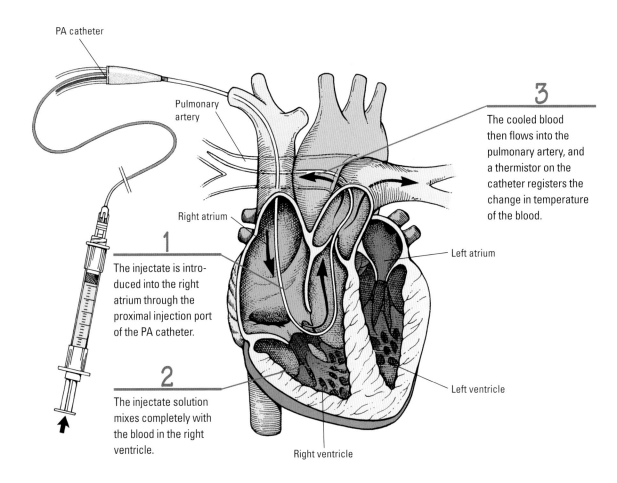

PA catheter

Pulmonary artery

3

The cooled blood then flows into the pulmonary artery, and a thermistor on the catheter registers the change in temperature of the blood.

Right atrium

Left atrium

1

The injectate is introduced into the right atrium through the proximal injection port of the PA catheter.

2

The injectate solution mixes completely with the blood in the right ventricle.

Left ventricle

Right ventricle

CCO pulmonary artery catheters have a heating filament in them, which heats the blood in the right ventricle, and the temperature change is sensed by the thermistor at the distal end of the catheter.

Analyzing thermodilution curves

The thermodilution curve provides valuable information about CO, injection technique, and equipment problems. When studying the curve, keep in mind that the area under the curve is inversely proportionate to CO: the smaller the area under the curve, the higher the CO; the larger the area under the curve, the lower the CO.

In addition to providing a record of CO, the curve may indicate problems related to technique, such as erratic or slow injectate instillations, or other problems, such as respiratory variations or electrical interference. The curves shown here correspond to those typically seen in clinical practice.

Normal thermodilution curve

In a patient who has adequate CO, the thermodilution curve begins with a smooth, rapid upstroke (representing proper injection technique) and is followed by a smooth, gradual downslope. The height of the curve varies, depending on whether you use a room temperature or an iced injectate.

Cardiac index
*Measurement of CO per unit of time that takes into account the patient's body surface area (BSA)
*Normally calculated in L/min/m^2
Cardiac index = CO ÷ BSA

Normal ranges
For nonpregnant adults: 2.5 to 4.2 L/min/m^2
For pregnant women: 3.5 to 6.5 L/min/m^2

High CO curve

A high CO curve has a rapid, smooth upstroke. Because the ventricles are ejecting blood too forcefully, the injectate moves through the heart quickly and the curve returns to baseline more rapidly. The smaller area under the curve suggests high CO.

Low CO curve

A low CO curve has a rapid, smooth upstroke. However, because blood is being ejected less efficiently from the ventricles, the injectate warms slowly and takes longer to be ejected. Consequently, the curve takes longer to return to baseline. This slow return produces a larger area under the curve, corresponding to low CO.

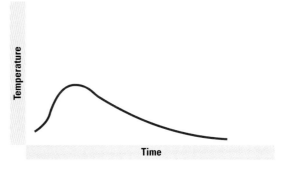

APCO monitoring

In APCO monitoring, a patient's existing arterial catheter is used to continuously calculate and display CO. It helps to determine a patient's fluid status and potential response to a fluid challenge before significant changes in blood pressure occur.

> The arterial catheter and line connect to a sensor, transducer, and monitor.

memory board

Important equations:

CO = Stroke volume × Heart rate
(normal CO is 4–8 L/min)

Pulse pressure = Systolic
pressure – Diastolic pressure

> The sensor measures variations in the patient's systolic and diastolic blood pressures to calculate pulse pressure, which is proportional to stroke volume (the volume of blood ejected by the ventricle with each contraction). Stroke volume and heart rate determine CO.

> The patient's age, gender, height, and weight are entered into a computer and are used to determine vascular compliance and resistance.

Pulse oximetry monitoring

Performed intermittently or continuously, pulse oximetry is a simple procedure used to noninvasively monitor arterial oxygen saturation. Two light-
emitting diodes (LEDs) send red and infrared light through a pulsating
arterial vascular bed, commonly in the fingertip or earlobe. A photodetector
measures the transmitted light as it passes through the vascular bed, detects
the relative amount of color absorbed by arterial blood, and calculates the
exact arterial oxygen saturation.

Arterial oxygen saturation values
obtained by pulse oximetry are
indicated by the symbol SpO_2,
whereas invasively measured arterial
oxygen saturation values are
indicated by the symbol SaO_2.

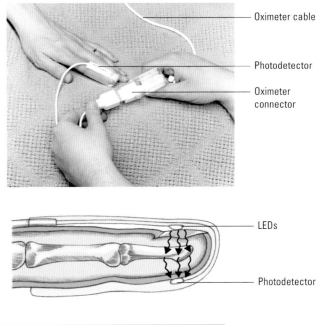

Oximeter cable

Photodetector

Oximeter
connector

LEDs

Photodetector

Oximeter monitor

Able to label?

Label each component of the normal arterial waveform shown here.

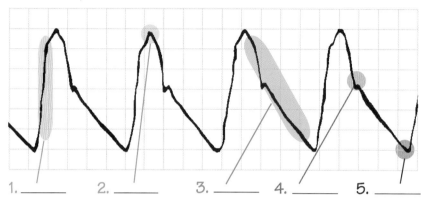

1. _____ 2. _____ 3. _____ 4. _____ 5. _____

Matchmaker

Match the abnormal arterial waveforms shown to their possible causes.

1.

2.

3.

4.

5.

6.

A. Pulsus paradoxus

B. Ventilator

C. Pulsus alternans

D. Ventricular bigeminy

E. Aortic stenosis

F. Overdamped waveform

Answers: Able to label? 1. Anacrotic limb, 2. Systolic peak, 3. Dicrotic limb, 4. Dicrotic notch, 5. End diastole; Matchmaker: 1. B, 2. D, 3. A, 4. F, 5. C, 6. E.

Suggested References

Cecconi, M., et al. Consensus on Circulatory Shock and Hemodynamic Monitoring. Task Force of the European Society of Intensive Care Medicine, *Intensive Care Medicine* 40:1795–1815, 2014. doi:10.1007/s00134-014-3525-z

Cronhjort, M., et al. Impact of Hemodynamic Goal-Directed Resuscitation on Mortality in Adult Critically Ill Patients: A Systematic Review and Meta-Analysis, *Journal of Clinical Monitoring and Computing* 2017. doi:10.1007/s10877-017-0032-0

Furer, A., Wessler, J., & Burkhoff, D. Hemodynamics of Cardiogenic Shock, *Interventional Cardiology Clinics* 16(3):359–371, 2017. doi:10.1016/j.iccl.2017.03.006

Magder, S. Invasive Hemodynamic Monitoring. *Critical Care Clinics* 31(1):67–87, 2015.

Chapter 6

Common disorders

Inflammatory disorders

Inflammatory cardiac disorders include endocarditis, myocarditis, and pericarditis. In patients with these conditions, scar formation and otherwise normal healing processes can cause debilitating structural damage to the heart.

Endocarditis

Endocarditis is an inflammation of the endocardium, the heart valves, or a cardiac prosthesis. It typically results from bacterial invasion and, therefore, may also be referred to as *infective endocarditis (IE)*. *Noninfective endocarditis* occurs when sterile blood clots develop on the valve in the absence of infection. It is often referred to as *nonbacterial thrombotic endocarditis* (NBTE).

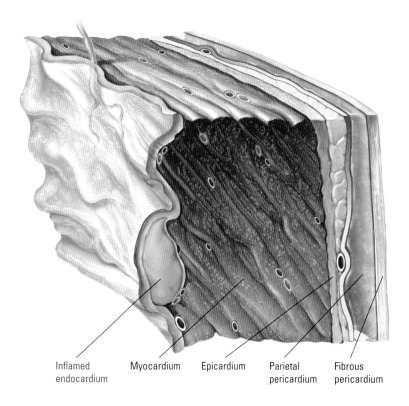

Inflamed endocardium   Myocardium   Epicardium   Parietal pericardium   Fibrous pericardium

Libman-Sacks endocarditis

Found in patients with systemic lupus erythematosus, Libman-Sacks endocarditis is characterized by wartlike vegetations on the leaflets of the mitral valve. It is an example of noninfective endocarditis.

Untreated endocarditis usually proves fatal. However, with proper treatment, the cure rate ranges from 60% to 98%.

Bacterial endocarditis

In bacterial endocarditis, the leaflets of the mitral valve erode and are eventually destroyed by bacterial invasion.

What's in a name?

The terminology used to describe IE changes as the causes of the disease become better understood. Some common names include:
- **acute bacterial endocarditis (ABE)** — describes a rapidly progressive disease process
- **subacute bacterial endocarditis (SBE)** — describes a disease process that lasts several months
- **rheumatic IE** — describes disease caused by rheumatic fever–related damage to heart valves
- **native valve IE** — affects original heart valves
- **prosthetic valve IE** — affects artificial heart valves
- **IVDA IE** — affects I.V. drug abusers
- **nosocomial IE** — describes disease that's associated with hospitalization.

Signs and symptoms of endocarditis

- Fever, chills, night sweats
- Fatigue, weight loss
- Cough, dyspnea, orthopnea
- Signs and symptoms of stroke/TIA
- New murmur or a change in existing murmur
- Petechiae
- Osler's nodes
- Janeway's lesions
- Splinter hemorrhages

Treatment of endocarditis seeks to eradicate the infecting organisms. Common organisms include staphylococci, especially *S. aureus*; streptococci; and *Candida albicans*.

Rx
- I.V. antibiotics
- Oral antibiotics
- Corrective surgery

Myocarditis

Myocarditis is focal or diffuse inflammation of the cardiac muscle (myocardium). It can be acute, subacute, or chronic and can occur at any age.

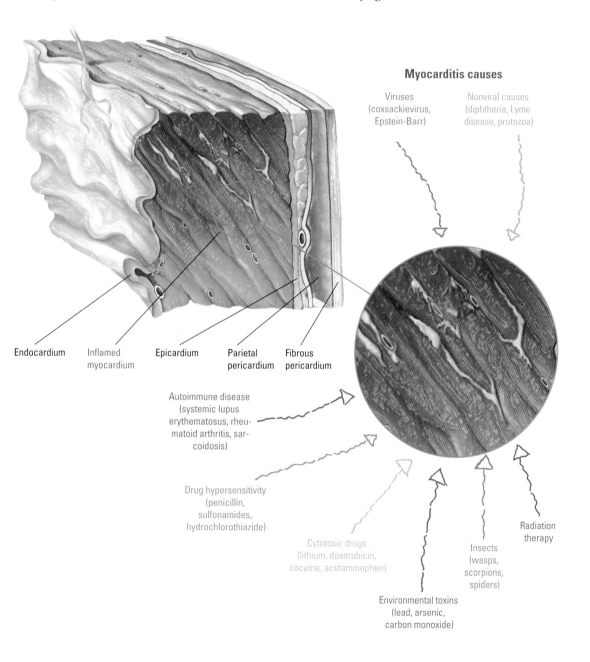

Myocarditis causes

Viruses
(coxsackievirus,
Epstein-Barr)

Nonviral causes
(diphtheria, Lyme
disease, protozoa)

Endocardium   Inflamed   Epicardium   Parietal   Fibrous
               myocardium   pericardium   pericardium

Autoimmune disease
(systemic lupus
erythematosus, rheu-
matoid arthritis, sar-
coidosis)

Drug hypersensitivity
(penicillin,
sulfonamides,
hydrochlorothiazide)

Cytotoxic drugs
(lithium, doxorubicin,
cocaine, acetaminophen)

Radiation
therapy

Insects
(wasps,
scorpions,
spiders)

Environmental toxins
(lead, arsenic,
carbon monoxide)

Viral myocarditis

Viral infections are the most common cause of myocarditis in the United States.

Lymphocytes and macrophages invade the myocardial muscle fibers, force them apart, and disrupt their normal function.

Normal myocardial fibers

Signs and symptoms of myocarditis

- Dyspnea on exertion and fatigue
- Palpitations
- Viral symptoms (fever, chills, myalgias)
- Mild, continuous pressure or soreness in the chest
- Signs and symptoms of heart failure (with severe disease)

Usually...

Myocarditis fails to produce specific cardiovascular symptoms or ECG abnormalities. The patient commonly experiences spontaneous recovery without residual defects.

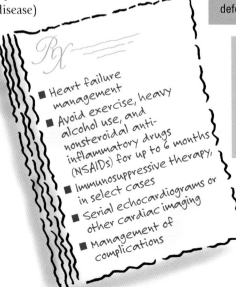

Rx

- Heart failure management
- Avoid exercise, heavy alcohol use, and nonsteroidal anti-inflammatory drugs (NSAIDs) for up to 6 months
- Immunosuppressive therapy, in select cases
- Serial echocardiograms or other cardiac imaging
- Management of complications

Sometimes...

The myocardium becomes damaged. As a result, arrhythmias, left-sided heart enlargement, and scarring can occur, but these problems can usually be readily managed.

Rarely...

Myocarditis is complicated by heart failure and leads to cardiomyopathy or arrhythmia-related death.

Pericarditis

Pericarditis is an inflammation of the pericardium. Most cases are considered idiopathic and are presumed to be viral. Other causes of pericarditis include infection, inflammation, radiation therapy, trauma, renal failure, cancer, and myocardial infarction (MI).

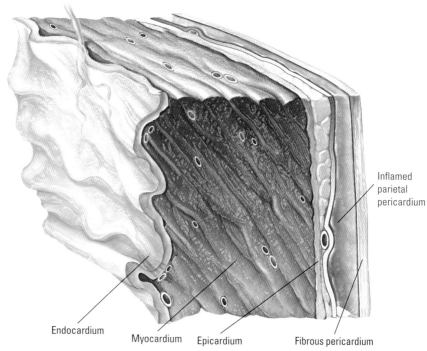

Inflamed parietal pericardium

Endocardium   Myocardium   Epicardium   Fibrous pericardium

The inflammatory process in pericarditis

1	2	3	4	5
Pericardial tissue damaged by bacteria or other substances releases chemical mediators of inflammation into the surrounding tissue.	Friction occurs as the inflamed pericardial layers rub against each other.	Histamines and other chemical mediators dilate vessels and increase vessel permeability.	Fluids and protein (including fibrinogen) leak into the tissues, causing extracellular edema. Macrophages, neutrophils, and monocytes in the tissue begin to phagocytose the invading bacteria.	Gradually, the space fills with an exudate composed of necrotic tissue, dead and dying bacteria, neutrophils, and macrophages. These products are eventually reabsorbed into healthy tissue.

Acute

Acute pericarditis can be fibrinous or effusive with purulent, serous, or hemorrhagic exudate. Buildup of fluid can cause pericardial effusion. If the effusion builds too rapidly, cardiac tamponade may occur.

Chronic

Chronic constrictive pericarditis is characterized by dense, fibrous pericardial thickening (shown below). This thickening causes constriction of normal heart size and movement, which can lead to permanently reduced stroke volume and cardiac output.

Signs and symptoms of acute pericarditis

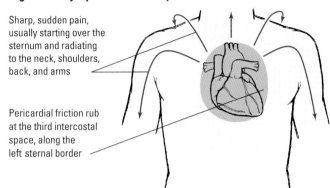

Sharp, sudden pain, usually starting over the sternum and radiating to the neck, shoulders, back, and arms

Pericardial friction rub at the third intercostal space, along the left sternal border

Signs and symptoms of chronic constrictive pericarditis

- Dyspnea
- Fatigue
- Chest pain with exertion
- Inspiratory jugular vein distention (Kussmaul's sign)
- Ascites and peripheral edema

Thick, fibrous pericardium

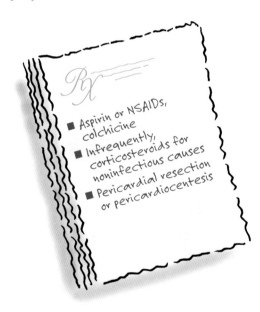

℞

- Aspirin or NSAIDs, colchicine
- Infrequently, corticosteroids for noninfectious causes
- Pericardial resection or pericardiocentesis

Valvular disorders

Valvular disease, which can occur in any of the heart valves, can be characterized as prolapse, insufficiency (regurgitation), or stenosis. It causes problems with opening and closing of the valves.

Possible causes

- Myxomatous degeneration (weakening with aging)
- Calcific degeneration
- IE
- Coronary artery disease (CAD)
- MI
- Connective tissue disorder

Potential complications

- Arrhythmias
- Cardiomyopathy
- Heart failure
- Thrombotic disorders

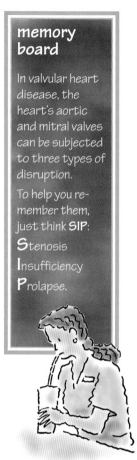

memory board

In valvular heart disease, the heart's aortic and mitral valves can be subjected to three types of disruption.

To help you remember them, just think **SIP**:

Stenosis
Insufficiency
Prolapse.

Mitral valve prolapse

Generally a benign disorder, mitral valve prolapse is often called *click-murmur syndrome* because of the auscultatory sounds commonly associated with it. Some patients complain of palpitations or chest pain.

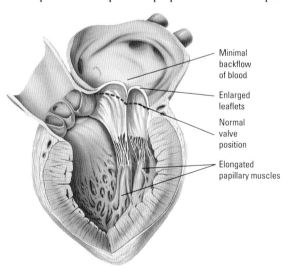

- Minimal backflow of blood
- Enlarged leaflets
- Normal valve position
- Elongated papillary muscles

Rx

- Elimination of caffeine and alcohol
- Smoking cessation
- Antiarrhythmic medications, if needed

Mitral insufficiency

Mitral insufficiency, also called *mitral regurgitation*, occurs when the mitral valve doesn't close completely, allowing blood to flow back through the valve.

1

Blood from the left ventricle flows back into the left atrium during systole, causing the atrium to enlarge to accommodate the backflow.

2

As a result, the left ventricle dilates to accommodate the increased blood volume from the atrium and to compensate for diminished cardiac output.

3

Ventricular hypertrophy and increased backpressure in the left atrium result in increased pulmonary artery pressure, eventually leading to left-sided and right-sided heart failure.

Increased left atrial pressure

Aortic valve

Leaking mitral valve

Abnormal backflow of blood

Normal direction of blood flow

Left ventricular dilation

You'll hear a holosystolic murmur if you listen at the apex of the heart.

Acute

Acute mitral insufficiency can start suddenly, with the characteristic sign being severe dyspnea.

Chronic

Chronic mitral insufficiency is a slow process that's accompanied by symptoms such as fatigue and insomnia.

Signs and symptoms

- Orthopnea or dyspnea
- Fatigue
- Angina and palpitations
- New-onset atrial fibrillation
- Systolic murmur

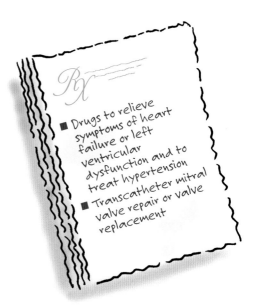

Mitral valve stenosis

Mitral valve stenosis is hardening of the mitral valve caused by fibrosis or calcification. This hardening results in narrowing of the valve opening, which obstructs blood flow from the left atrium to the left ventricle. Consequently, left atrial volume and pressure increase, and the chamber dilates.

Mitral stenosis typically occurs in females. It most commonly results from rheumatic fever and may also be associated with congenital anomalies.

Pulmonary hypertension develops

Left atrium dilation

Narrowed mitral valve

Lung congestion and pressure

Right-sided heart failure

Signs and symptoms

- Dyspnea on exertion (DOE), paroxysmal nocturnal dyspnea (PND), and orthopnea
- Fatigue and weakness
- Right-sided heart failure (HF) and cardiac arrhythmias
- Crackles on auscultation

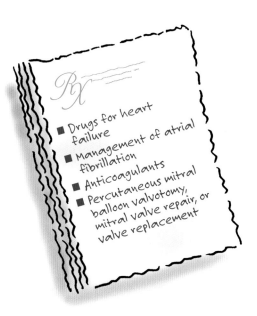

Aortic insufficiency

Aortic insufficiency, or aortic regurgitation, occurs when the aortic semilunar valve doesn't close completely. In this condition, blood flows back through the valve into the left ventricle. It can result from rheumatic fever, syphilis, hypertension, or endocarditis, or it may be idiopathic. It's also associated with Marfan's syndrome and with ventricular septal defect, even after surgical closure.

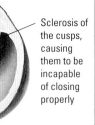

Oh boy. Aortic insufficiency typically occurs in males.

Aortic valve

Left ventricle

Sclerosis of the cusps, causing them to be incapable of closing properly

Signs and symptoms

- Exertional dyspnea
- Orthopnea and paroxysmal nocturnal dyspnea (PND)
- Cough
- Left-sided heart failure
- Pulsus bisferiens (rapidly rising and collapsing pulses)
- Blowing diastolic murmur or S_3

A sign by any other name. . .

Many common signs seen in aortic insufficiency have been named after the physicians who first documented them. Here are a few for you to spot.

Sign	Description
de Musset's sign	Bobbing of the head with every pulse
Hill's sign	Blood pressure that's higher in the arms than in the legs
Quincke's sign	Pulsatile flushing and blanching of the fingernail bed with gentle pressure
Traube's sign	Pistol-shot–like sound auscultated over the femoral arteries

The role of drug therapy in severe aortic insufficiency is limited to symptomatic patients or asymptomatic patients with LV systolic dysfunction who are not candidates for aortic valve surgery.

CAUTION

Rx

- Valve replacement
- Drugs to treat diastolic hypertension
- Drug therapy in preparation for aortic valve surgery

Aortic stenosis

Aortic stenosis (AS) results from a congenital bicuspid aortic valve with super-imposed calcification, calcification of a normal trileaflet valve, or rheumatic disease.

4

Diminished cardiac output causes poor coronary artery perfusion, ischemia of the left ventricle, and left-sided heart failure.

1

The aortic valve or the aorta hardens, and the valvular opening narrows.

2

Left ventricular pressure rises to overcome the resistance of the narrowed valve.

Elderly patients are at increased risk for aortic stenosis due to atherosclerosis.

3

Oxygen demand increases with the added workload.

Signs and symptoms

Early symptoms
- Exertional dyspnea or decreased exercise tolerance
- Syncope, presyncope, or exertional dizziness
- Exertional angina

Classic or end-stage symptoms
- Angina
- Left-sided heart failure
- Syncope

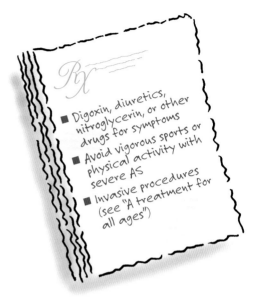

- Digoxin, diuretics, nitroglycerin, or other drugs for symptoms
- Avoid vigorous sports or physical activity with severe AS
- Invasive procedures (see "A treatment for all ages")

A treatment for all ages

In children who don't have calcified valves, simple commissurotomy under direct visualization is usually effective.

Adults with calcified valves need valve replacement when they become symptomatic or are at risk for developing left-sided heart failure.

Transcatheter aortic valve replacement is an option for severe AS, especially in those patients who are at a prohibitive or very high surgical risk. Alternatively, balloon aortic valvotomy procedure may be reasonable as a bridge to surgery in unstable patients or as palliative therapy.

Degenerative disorders

Degenerative disorders, which cause damage over time, are the most common cardiovascular ailments. The onset of these disorders may be insidious, triggering symptoms only after the disease has progressed.

Hypertension

Hypertension (HTN) refers to intermittent or sustained elevation in diastolic or systolic blood pressure (BP).

Types of hypertension and their causes

Essential (primary, idiopathic)
- Caused by complex abnormalities in the mechanisms that control cardiac output, systemic vascular resistance, and blood volume
- More than 90% of all cases

Causes
- Environmental factors, such as obesity, stress, and high salt intake
- Genetic factors, such as insulin resistance
- Increased sympathetic nervous system activity

Secondary
- Caused by another disorder
- Accounts for less than 10% of all cases

Causes
- Renovascular diseases or primary kidney disease
- Primary aldosteronism or Cushing's syndrome
- Congenital coarctation (narrowing) of the aorta
- Drugs, such as hormonal contraceptives, NSAIDs, over-the-counter (OTC) stimulants
- Sleep apnea
- Pheochromocytoma

Signs and symptoms

- Increased BP measurements on two or more readings taken at two or more visits after an initial screening
- Headaches
- Retinal changes
- Evidence of disease causing secondary hypertension
- Complications of sustained elevation

Malignant hypertension is a rare, severe form of hypertension that's characterized by a BP of 220/120 mm Hg or more.

Blood pressure classifications

BP is also classified based on the degree of elevation of the readings. This table classifies blood pressure according to systolic blood pressure (SBP) and diastolic blood pressure (DBP).

BP classification	Normal	Prehypertension	Stage 1	Stage 2
SBP (mm Hg)	< 120	120 to 139	140 to 159	≥ 160
	and	or	or	or
DBP (mm Hg)	<80	80 to 89	90 to 99	≥ 100

The silent killer

Although patients may feel healthy, untreated or poorly controlled hypertension can be damaging to their major organs.

Brain

Stroke

Stroke from blood clots in narrowed blood vessels or from hemorrhage of a weakened vessel wall (aneurysm) can be disabling or fatal.

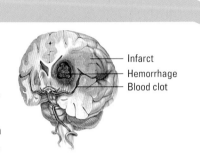

- Infarct
- Hemorrhage
- Blood clot

Eye

Hypertensive retinopathy

Effects on the blood vessels within the retina can lead to hemorrhage, hard exudate, and swelling of the optic disc that may result in blindness.

- Cotton-wool spot
- Flame-shaped hemorrhage
- Swollen optic disk
- Hard exudates

Retina

Heart

Myocardial infarction (MI)

MI may result from atherosclerosis of the coronary arteries.

Aneurysm

Increased blood pressure causes blood vessels to weaken and bulge, forming an aneurysm. A ruptured aneurysm can be fatal.

Heart failure

Kidney

Nephrosclerosis

Arterioles in the kidney harden and restrict oxygenation of the glomeruli, causing scarring and kidney failure.

Glomerulus

Preventing pressure problems

Preventing the onset of hypertension is the first goal of the Joint National Committee on Prevention, Detection, Evaluation, and Treatment of High Blood Pressure. Evidence shows that lifestyle interventions, such as those listed here, are critical to meeting this goal:
• increasing exercise
• consuming a DASH diet (rich in fruits, vegetables, low-fat dairy) low in salt and fat
• maintaining a healthy body weight and a body mass index (BMI, 18.5 to 24.9 kg/m^2)
• limiting alcohol intake.

℞
■ Lifestyle changes
■ Thiazide-type diuretics, calcium channel blockers, ACE inhibitors, or ARBs
■ Tobacco cessation

Pulmonary hypertension

Pulmonary hypertension refers to chronically elevated pulmonary artery pressure (PAP) of 25 mm Hg or greater at rest as measured by right heart catheterization.

There are two types of pulmonary hypertension:
• In *primary*, or *idiopathic*, pulmonary hypertension, the intimal linings of the pulmonary arteries thicken, narrowing the lumen and increasing vascular resistance. No cause is known.
• *Secondary* pulmonary hypertension begins with diseases that cause alveolar destruction or prevent the chest wall from expanding sufficiently.

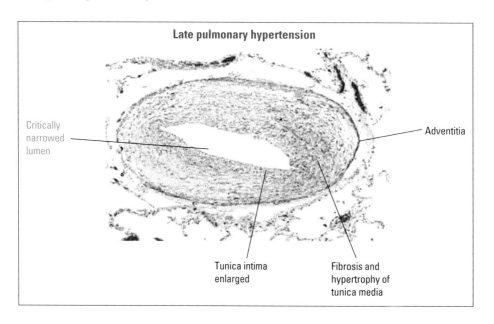

Late pulmonary hypertension

Critically narrowed lumen

Adventitia

Tunica intima enlarged

Fibrosis and hypertrophy of tunica media

What happens?

Pulmonary hypertension can be caused by a number of factors, all of which force the heart's right side to work harder to pump blood to the lungs. The right chambers may enlarge as they struggle to function, and blood is often forced backward through the tricuspid valve.

Signs and symptoms

- Exertional dyspnea, weakness, syncope, and fatigue
- Tachycardia
- Decreased BP
- Tachypnea with mild exertion
- Peripheral edema, ascites, jugular vein distention (JVD), and hepatomegaly
- Easily palpable right ventricular lift and a reduced carotid pulse

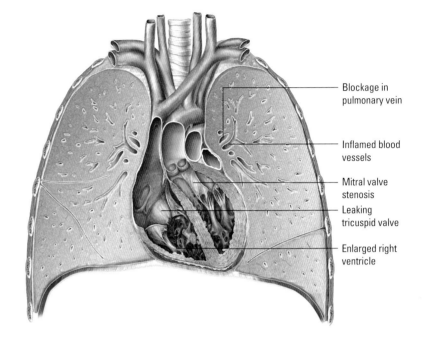

- Blockage in pulmonary vein
- Inflamed blood vessels
- Mitral valve stenosis
- Leaking tricuspid valve
- Enlarged right ventricle

Sorry for the noise, folks. We're experiencing a little turbulence.

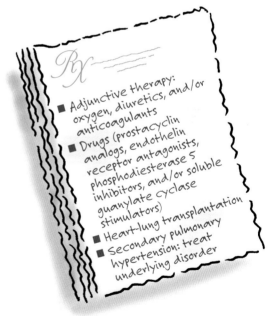

℞

- Adjunctive therapy: oxygen, diuretics, and/or anticoagulants
- Drugs (prostacyclin analogs, endothelin receptor antagonists, phosphodiesterase 5 inhibitors, and/or soluble guanylate cyclase stimulators)
- Heart-lung transplantation
- Secondary pulmonary hypertension: treat underlying disorder

Heart failure

Heart failure (HF) occurs when the myocardium can't pump effectively enough to meet the body's metabolic needs. A complex interaction of the factors listed here leads to the syndrome of heart failure:

- altered myocardial function due to increased pressure or volume within the heart
- left ventricular remodeling, with initial hypertrophy and then severe dilation
- altered hemodynamics that result from an effort to maintain cardiac output despite increased diastolic filling pressure
- neurohormonal changes that accelerate heart rate and initially increase ejection fraction and then trigger a local inflammatory response that becomes systemic in severe disease.

They say I'm a failure! But it's not my fault.

Left ventricular hypertrophy

Hypertrophy of the left ventricle is one of the heart's first steps to compensate for either increased pressures or increased blood volume.

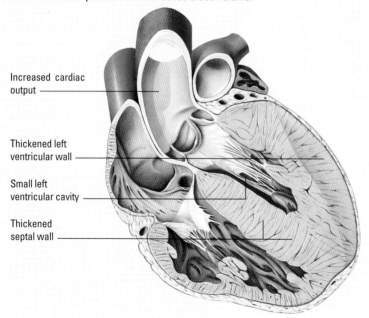

Increased cardiac output

Thickened left ventricular wall

Small left ventricular cavity

Thickened septal wall

A Starling named Frank?

The Frank-Starling law says that the amount of cardiac muscle stretch correlates directly with the force of contraction. This accounts for the heart's ability to pump more blood during exertion in addition to its ability to compensate for sustained abnormal increases in blood volume.

Frank

Three ways to classify heart failure

Heart failure can be classified according to its pathophysiology. It may be right sided or left sided, systolic or diastolic, and acute or chronic.

1

Right sided or left sided

Right-sided heart failure is the result of ineffective right ventricular contraction. It may be caused by an acute right ventricular infarction or pulmonary embolus. However, the most common cause is profound backward blood flow due to left-sided heart failure.

   Left-sided heart failure is the result of ineffective left ventricular contraction. It may lead to pulmonary congestion or pulmonary edema and decreased cardiac output. Left ventricular MI, hypertension, and aortic or mitral valve stenosis or insufficiency are common causes. As the left ventricle's decreased pumping ability persists, fluid accumulates, backing up into the left atrium, then into the lungs. If this worsens, pulmonary edema and right-sided heart failure may also result.

2

Systolic or diastolic

In systolic heart failure, the left ventricle can't pump enough blood out to the systemic circulation during systole, and the ejection fraction falls. Consequently, blood backs up into the pulmonary circulation, pressure rises in the pulmonary venous system, and cardiac output falls.

   In diastolic heart failure, the left ventricle can't relax and fill properly during diastole, and the stroke volume falls. Therefore, larger ventricular volumes are needed to maintain cardiac output.

3

Acute or chronic

The term *acute* refers to the timing of the onset of symptoms and whether compensatory mechanisms kick in. Typically, in acute heart failure, fluid status is normal or low, and sodium and water retention don't occur.

   In chronic heart failure, signs and symptoms have been present for some time, compensatory mechanisms have taken effect, and fluid volume overload persists. Drugs, diet changes, and activity restrictions usually control symptoms.

Signs and symptoms of right-sided failure

- Edema, initially dependent
- Jugular vein distention
- Hepatomegaly
- Ascites
- Generalized weight gain
- Weakness

Who knew my split personality could have such an effect on the body?

Signs and symptoms of left-sided failure

- Dyspnea, initially on exertion
- Cough
- Tachycardia
- Fatigue
- Muscle weakness
- Cyanosis or pallor
- Bibasilar crackles

Photo op

Looking for edema

Compare one foot and leg with the other, noting their relative size and the prominence of veins, tendons, and bones. Note that edema may obscure these features. Edema can be pitting or nonpitting.

All landmarks visible

Decreased visibility of veins and bony prominences

Normal   **Edematous**

Pitting edema

"Pitting" is a result of the inelasticity of fluid-filled tissue. To differentiate pitting edema from nonpitting edema, press your finger against a swollen area for 5 seconds and then quickly remove it. If the indentation fills slowly, pitting edema is present. To determine the severity of pitting edema, estimate the indentation's depth in centimeters: +1 (1 cm), +2 (2 cm), +3 (3 cm), or +4 (4 cm).

Pitting edema

Classifying signs and symptoms to determine treatment

Two sets of guidelines are available to help direct treatment of patients with heart failure. The New York Heart Association (NYHA) classification is based on functional capacity. The American College of Cardiology/American Heart Association (ACC/AHA) guidelines are based on objective assessment. These guidelines are compared side-by-side below.

NYHA classification	ACC/AHA guidelines	Recommendations
	Stage A: Patient at high risk for developing heart failure but without structural heart disease or signs and symptoms of heart failure	• Treatment of hypertension, lipid disorders, and diabetes • Smoking cessation and regular exercise • Discouraged use of alcohol and illicit drugs • Angiotensin-converting enzyme inhibitor (ACEI) or ARB, if indicated
Class I: Ordinary physical activity doesn't cause undue fatigue, palpitations, dyspnea, or angina.	*Stage B:* Structural heart disease without signs and symptoms of heart failure	• All stage A therapies • ACEI or ARB (as appropriate) • Beta-adrenergic blocker (as appropriate) • Select patients: implantable cardioverter-defibrillator (ICD), revascularization, or valve surgery
Class II: Patient has slight limitation of physical activity but is asymptomatic at rest. Ordinary physical activity causes fatigue, palpitations, dyspnea, or anginal pain. *Class III:* Patient has marked limitation of physical activity but is typically asymptomatic at rest. Less than ordinary physical activity causes fatigue, palpitations, dyspnea, or angina.	*Stage C:* Structural heart disease with prior or current signs and symptoms of heart failure *HFrEF:* Heart failure with reduced ejection fraction (EF 40% or lower) *HFpEF:* Heart failure with preserved ejection fraction (EF 50% or greater)	• All stage A and B therapies *HFrEF:* • ACEI or ARB or ARNI (angiotensin receptor-neprilysin inhibitor) ***AND*** Beta-blocker • Aldosterone antagonists • Diuretics • Select patients: ivabradine, hydralnitrates, and/or digoxin • Avoiding or withdrawing antiarrhythmic agents, most calcium channel blockers, and NSAIDs *HFpEF:* • Blood pressure control • Diuretics to treat symptoms • Treat comorbidities
Class IV: Patient is unable to perform any physical activity without discomfort; symptoms may be present at rest. Discomfort increases with physical activity.	*Stage D:* End-stage disease requiring specialized treatment strategies, such as mechanical circulatory support, continuous inotropic infusion, or heart transplantation	• All therapies for stages A, B, and C • Heart transplantation • Mechanical left ventricular assist device • Continuous inotropic therapy • Hospice care

A smaller "Dor"

The Dor procedure, also called *partial left ventriculectomy* or *ventricular remodeling*, involves the removal of nonviable heart muscle to reduce the size of the hypertrophied ventricle, thereby allowing the heart to pump more efficiently. This procedure isn't indicated for all patients, though.

Rx
■ Treatment of underlying disorders
■ Lifestyle changes to decrease effects
■ Drugs per protocol above
■ Cardiac resynchronization therapy, implantable cardioverter-defibrillator, or heart transplantation

Cardiomyopathy

Cardiomyopathy generally refers to disease of the heart muscle fibers. It takes three main forms.

Dilated cardiomyopathy

Dilated cardiomyopathy primarily affects systolic function. Here's what happens:

Secondary increased atrial chamber size

Increased ventricular chamber size (dilation)

Decreased muscle size, but increased heart size

The pathophysiology steps

Step 1

Cardiac muscle fibers are extensively damaged.

Step 2

Contractility in the left ventricle decreases, lowering stroke volume.

Step 3

Early changes of heart failure (increased heart rate and left ventricular hypertrophy) help the heart to compensate functionally.

Step 4

The compensatory mechanisms eventually are unable to maintain adequate cardiac output.

Step 5

Severe left ventricular dilation occurs as venous return and systemic vascular resistance increase.

Step 6

Eventually, all chambers may dilate, causing generalized cardiomegaly with associated risk of arrhythmias and emboli.

Signs and symptoms

- Shortness of breath, orthopnea, dyspnea on exertion, paroxysmal nocturnal dyspnea, fatigue, and a dry cough at night caused by left-sided heart failure
- Peripheral edema, hepatomegaly, jugular vein distention, and weight gain caused by right-sided heart failure
- Tachycardia with irregular pulse, if atrial fibrillation exists
- Pansystolic murmur associated with mitral and tricuspid insufficiency

For a patient with dilated cardiomyopathy, signs and symptoms may be overlooked until left-sided heart failure occurs. Evaluate the patient's current condition and then compare it with his or her condition over the past 6 to 12 months.

Rx
- Treatment of underlying disorders
- Lifestyle modifications to increase functional capacity
- ACE inhibitors or ARBs or ARNI (angiotensin receptor-neprilysin inhibitor)
- Drugs to treat heart failure and arrhythmias
- Cardiomyoplasty or heart transplantation

Hypertrophic cardiomyopathy

Hypertrophic cardiomyopathy primarily affects diastolic function. Here's what happens:

Obstructive hypertrophic cardiomyopathy is almost always inherited as a non–sex-linked autosomal dominant trait.

Increased pulmonary vascular pressure

Mitral insufficiency due to hypertrophy of papillary muscles and septum

Failure of left ventricle to relax properly, slowing diastolic filling

Thickened interventricular septum that may obstruct blood flow to the aortic valve

Left ventricular hypertrophy and stiffening

Small intramural coronary arteries that can't supply the necessary oxygen to the enlarged cardiac muscle, resulting in angina or ischemia

Signs and symptoms

- Syncope or sudden cardiac death (commonly the presenting symptom)
- Angina
- Dyspnea
- Fatigue
- Pulse irregularities
- Systolic ejection murmur along the left sternal border and apex

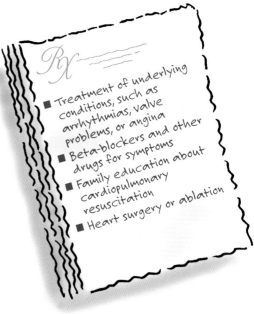

Rx

- Treatment of underlying conditions, such as arrhythmias, valve problems, or angina
- Beta-blockers and other drugs for symptoms
- Family education about cardiopulmonary resuscitation
- Heart surgery or ablation

Restrictive cardiomyopathy

Restrictive cardiomyopathy is characterized by stiffness of the ventricle caused by left ventricular hypertrophy and endocardial fibrosis and thickening. Here's what happens:

Decreased cardiac output with high diastolic pressure compared to the amount of diastolic volume

Enlarged atria due to rigid ventricular walls, causing atrial fibrillation

Failure of the left ventricle to relax properly, slowing diastolic filling

Left ventricular hypertrophy

Ventricular rigidity from fibrosis that impairs contraction during systole

Incompetent atrioventricular valves, allowing backward flow of blood

Decreased ventricular chamber size from endocardial fibrosis and thickening

Signs and symptoms

- Fatigue
- Dyspnea
- Orthopnea
- Chest pain
- Edema
- Liver engorgement
- High systemic and pulmonary venous pressure

Keep an eye out: restrictive cardiomyopathy can resemble constrictive pericarditis.

Rx
- Treatment of underlying causes
- Diuretics, corticosteroids, positive intropic agents, or anticoagulants
- Fluid restriction
- Oxygen therapy
- Heart transplantation

Coronary artery disease

CAD results from the progressive buildup of atherosclerotic plaque in the coronary arteries.

The law of supply and demand

I demand some oxygen on my side, too. Pumping oxygenated blood throughout the body is hard work!

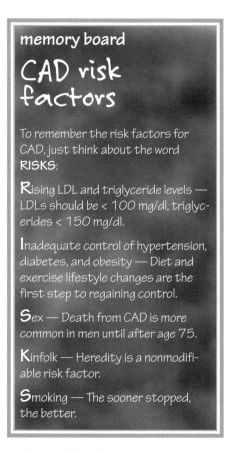

memory board

CAD risk factors

To remember the risk factors for CAD, just think about the word **RISKS**:

Rising LDL and triglyceride levels — LDLs should be < 100 mg/dl, triglycerides < 150 mg/dl.

Inadequate control of hypertension, diabetes, and obesity — Diet and exercise lifestyle changes are the first step to regaining control.

Sex — Death from CAD is more common in men until after age 75.

Kinfolk — Heredity is a nonmodifiable risk factor.

Smoking — The sooner stopped, the better.

Coronary artery close-up

Coronary arteries are normally flexible and can adapt to the oxygen-carrying needs of the heart.

— Tunica adventitia

— Tunica media

— Tunica intima

— Lumen

Understanding atherosclerosis

Atherosclerosis causes a buildup of fatty fibrous plaque in the vessel walls. Thrombi can also form if the plaque ruptures through the intimal layer. The lumen becomes increasingly narrow.

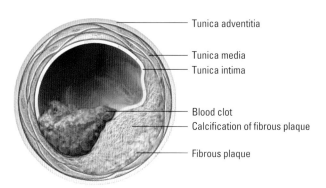

— Tunica adventitia

— Tunica media
— Tunica intima

— Blood clot
— Calcification of fibrous plaque

— Fibrous plaque

Signs and symptoms
- Possibly none
- Abnormal stress or echocardiogram findings
- Angina, typically with exertion or stress
- Major complications, such as acute coronary syndrome, heart failure, arrhythmias, or sudden death

Did you know I can cause mitral insufficiency and cardiomyopathy, too?

Stable angina

Angina is the classic sign of CAD. Stable angina can come in three forms: Prinzmetal's (variant) angina, microvascular (cardiac syndrome X) angina, and chronic stable angina.

Partially blocked artery, causing chronic stable angina

Capillary constriction, causing microvascular angina without blockage of coronary arteries

Area of vasospasm, causing Prinzmetal's angina

Prinzmetal's (variant) angina
- Characterized by resting discomfort, which can cause the patient to awaken at night and persists for hours
- Causes reversible ST-segment elevation during event
- Caused by coronary artery vasospasm
- Treated with calcium channel blockers alone or with long-acting nitrates, possibly beta-blockers, or coronary stenting/revascularization if intractable

Microvascular (cardiac syndrome X) angina
- Characterized by stable, angina-like chest pain
- Caused by damaged or diseased lining walls of small coronary arteries
- Poses no risk of cardiac ischemia because the capillaries are too small to block oxygenation of cardiac cells
- Treated by reducing cardiac risk factors and possible medications (nitrates, beta-blockers, calcium channel blockers, ACEI, or ARBs)

Chronic stable angina
- Characterized by exertional, rest-relieved discomfort located anywhere between the umbilicus and the ears that may be associated with numbness of the arms or hands
- Doesn't increase in frequency or severity over time
- Generally caused by fixed obstructive atheromatous lesions
- Treated with rest and nitrates; beta-blockers for prevention

Acute coronary syndromes

Patients with acute coronary syndromes (ACS) have some degree of coronary artery occlusion. Development begins with a rupture or erosion of plaque — an unstable and lipid-rich substance.

The rupture results in platelet adhesions, fibrin clot formation, and activation of thrombin.

A thrombus progresses and obstructs blood flow. (An early thrombus doesn't necessarily block blood flow.) The effect is an imbalance in myocardial oxygen supply and demand. Depending on the degree of occlusion, ACS is defined as three types.

If the patient has unstable angina, a thrombus partially occludes a coronary vessel. This thrombus is full of platelets. The partially occluded vessel may have distal microthrombi that cause necrosis in some myocytes.

If smaller vessels infarct, the patient is at higher risk for MI, which may progress to a non–ST-segment elevation MI. Usually, only the innermost layer of the heart is damaged.

ST-segment elevation MI results when reduced blood flow through one of the coronary arteries causes myocardial ischemia, injury, and necrosis. The damage extends through all myocardial layers.

ACS tissue destruction

The destruction of healthy cardiac tissue from myocardial ischemia varies with the severity of the ACS involved and the promptness of effective diagnosis and treatment.

Unstable angina means chest discomfort that's new, severe, or more frequent than three times daily. The ECG may be normal or show changes possibly indicating infarction, but cardiac biomarkers remain within normal limits.

Superior vena cava

Right atrial auricle

Right coronary artery

Arch of aorta

Pulmonary trunk

Left atrial auricle

Circumflex branch of left coronary artery

Left anterior descending artery

Papillary muscle

Damaged muscle from MI

Zones of MI

Reversible ischemia

Severe ischemia (recovery possible with revascularization)

Necrosis

Comparing signs and symptoms: unstable angina and MI

	Unstable angina	Myocardial infarction
Character, location, and radiation	• Burning, squeezing, substernal or retrosternal pain spreading across chest; may radiate to inside of arm, neck, jaw, or shoulder blade	• Severe, persistent substernal pain or pain over pericardium; may spread widely throughout chest and be accompanied by pain in shoulders and hands; may be described as crushing or squeezing
Duration of pain	• 5 to 15 min	• > 15 min
Precipitating events	• Usually related to exertion, emotion, eating, cold	• Occurs spontaneously • May be sequela to unstable angina
Relieving measures	• Rest, nitroglycerin, oxygen	• Morphine sulfate, successful reperfusion of blocked coronary artery
Associated symptoms	• Shortness of breath • Dizziness • Nausea • Palpitations • Weakness • Cold sweat	• Feeling of impending doom • Fatigue • Nausea and vomiting • Shortness of breath • Cool extremities • Perspiration • Anxiety
Associated signs	• Hypotension or hypertension • Tachycardia or bradycardia	• Hypotension or hypertension • Palpable precordial pulse • Muffled heart sounds • Arrhythmias
Cardiac biomarkers	• Usually within normal range	• Elevated

Atypical chest pain in women

Women with CAD may experience classic chest pain, which may occur without any relationship to activity or stress. However, they also commonly experience atypical chest pain, vague chest pain, or a lack of chest pain.

Location, location, location

Whereas men tend to complain of crushing pain in the center of the chest, women are more likely to experience arm or shoulder pain; jaw, neck, or throat pain; toothache; back pain; or pain under the breastbone or in the stomach.

Other signs and symptoms women may experience include nausea or dizziness; shortness of breath; unexplained anxiety, weakness, or fatigue; palpitations; cold sweat; or pallor.

Any patient may experience atypical chest pain, but it's more common in women.

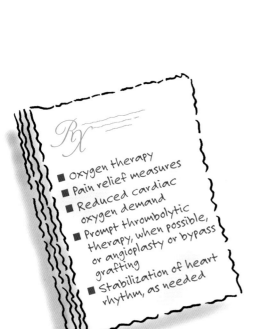

Rx

- Oxygen therapy
- Pain relief measures
- Reduced cardiac oxygen demand
- Prompt thrombolytic therapy, when possible, or angioplasty or bypass grafting
- Stabilization of heart rhythm, as needed

memory board

The American Heart Association's acronym for saying goodbye to heart disease, **ALOHA**, can help you remember recommendations for your female patients who are at risk:

Assess your risk. Know important levels, such as cholesterol, weight, and blood pressure.

Lifestyle is the priority. Lifestyle changes, such as smoking cessation, exercise, and a healthy diet, can help prevent cardiovascular disease.

Other interventions may be necessary if lifestyle changes don't significantly reduce the risk of heart disease. Consult a physician.

High-risk cases are serious and need to be addressed immediately and consistently.

Avoid hormone therapy, antioxidant vitamin supplements, and aspirin therapy because these treatments may do more harm than good, especially in low-risk patients.

Congenital disorders

Patent ductus arteriosus

The ductus arteriosus is a fetal blood vessel that connects the pulmonary artery to the descending aorta. Normally, the ductus closes within weeks after birth. However, with patent ductus arteriosus (PDA), it remains open, creating a left-to-right shunt of blood from the aorta to the pulmonary artery resulting in recirculation of arterial blood through the lungs. PDA is classified as an increased pulmonary blood flow defect.

Signs and symptoms

- Respiratory distress with signs of heart failure (in neonates)
- Gibson's murmur
- Wide pulse pressure
- Failure to thrive

Rx
- Diuretics and cardiac glycosides
- I.V. prostaglandin inhibitors
- Percutaneous closure with an occlusion device or with stainless steel coils
- Surgical closure during thoracotomy

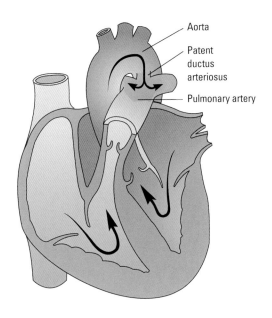

Aorta

Patent ductus arteriosus

Pulmonary artery

Atrial septal defect

An atrial septal defect (ASD) is an abnormal opening between the left and right atria. A small opening may cause few symptoms. However, if the opening is large, higher pressure in the left atrium can shunt large amounts of blood into the right atrium, which can result in right heart volume overload, right atrial and ventricular enlargement, and pulmonary hypertension. ASD is classified as an increased pulmonary blood flow defect and is one of the most common congenital heart defects.

Signs and symptoms

- Fatigue, dyspnea, exercise intolerance, palpitations, syncope
- Arrhythmias
- Early to midsystolic murmur; low-pitched diastolic murmur
- Fixed, widely split S_2
- Systolic click or late systolic murmur at the apex
- Clubbing of nails and cyanosis (with right-to-left shunt)
- Palpable pulsation of the pulmonary artery

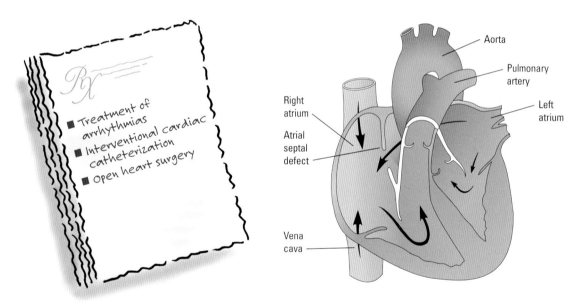

Ventricular septal defect

A ventricular septal defect (VSD), the most common type of congenital disorder, is an abnormal opening between the right and left ventricles that allows blood to shunt between them. Not always readily apparent at birth, the defect can be small and may close spontaneously, or the septum may be entirely absent, resulting in a single ventricle. A large, untreated defect can cause right ventricular hypertrophy, pulmonary hypertension, and heart failure. VSD is classified as an increased pulmonary blood flow defect.

Signs and symptoms

- Loud, harsh systolic murmur
- Fatigue
- Failure to thrive
- Cyanosis
- Clubbing
- Liver, heart, and spleen enlargement
- Diaphoresis
- Tachycardia
- Grunting respirations

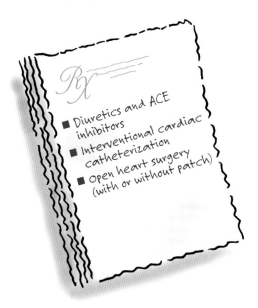

Rx
- Diuretics and ACE inhibitors
- Interventional cardiac catheterization
- Open heart surgery (with or without patch)

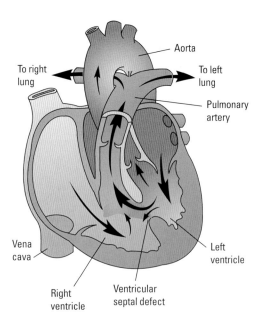

Coarctation of the aorta

Coarctation is a narrowing of the aorta, usually just below the left subclavian artery, near the site where the ligamentum arteriosum joins the pulmonary artery to the aorta. It can result from spasm and constriction of the smooth muscle in the ductus arteriosus as it closes. Restricted blood flow through the narrow aorta increases the pressure load on the left ventricle, resulting in dilation of the proximal aorta, left ventricle hypertrophy, elevated upper body blood pressures, and diminished blood flow to the lower body. The ductus arteriosus may be open or closed. Coarctation of the aorta is more common in boys and is the leading cause of heart failure in the first few months of life. It's classified as an obstruction to blood flow leaving the heart.

Signs and symptoms

- Heart failure
- Absent femoral pulses
- Blood pressure 20 mm Hg higher in the arms than in the legs
- Headache
- Vertigo
- Epistaxis

Rx

- Digoxin and diuretics
- Hypertension control with beta-blockers, ACEI, or ARBs
- Interventional balloon angiography
- Surgery

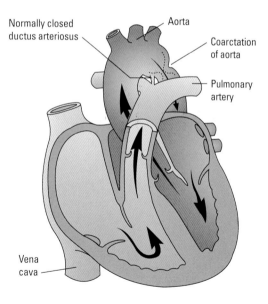

Normally closed ductus arteriosus

Aorta

Coarctation of aorta

Pulmonary artery

Vena cava

Vascular disorders

Vascular disorders can affect arteries, veins, or both. Arterial disorders include aneurysms, which result from weakening of the arterial wall, and arterial occlusive disease, which commonly results from atherosclerotic narrowing of the artery's lumen. Thrombophlebitis, a venous disorder, results from inflammation or occlusion of the affected vessel.

Aortic aneurysm

- Localized outpouching or abnormal dilation in a weakened arterial wall of the aorta.
- When developing, lateral pressure increases, causing the vessel lumen to widen and blood flow to slow.
- May result in hemodynamic forces that cause pulsatile stresses on the weakened wall and press on the small vessels that supply nutrients to the arterial wall, causing the aorta to become bowed and tortuous.

Signs and symptoms

- Possibly none when aneurysm is small (usually)
- Pain, hypotension, and decreased peripheral circulation when aneurysm is large, leaking, or pressing on internal structures
- Back pain, groin pain, and pulsating abdominal mass with rupture of abdominal aortic aneurysm

Locations of aortic aneurysms

- Syphilitic aneurysms are the common variety in the ascending aorta, which is usually spared by the atherosclerotic process.
- Atherosclerotic aneurysms usually occur in the abdominal aorta or iliac arteries.
- Mycotic aneurysms can occur anywhere that bacteria deposit on vessel walls.

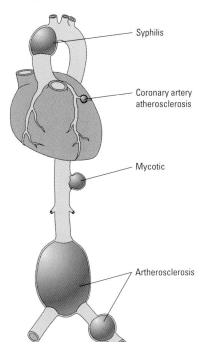

Syphilis

Coronary artery atherosclerosis

Mycotic

Artherosclerosis

An aortic aneurysm may suddenly rupture or tear, possibly causing death. Rupture of an aortic aneurysm is a medical emergency requiring prompt treatment.

Types

Saccular
A saccular aneurysm is an asymmetric outpouching of the arterial wall.

Aortic arch aneurysm

Fusiform
A fusiform aneurysm is a symmetrical spindle-shaped enlargement encompassing the entire aortic circumference.

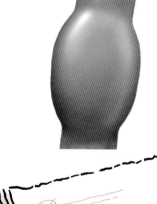

False
A false aneurysm occurs when the entire wall is injured, resulting in a break in all layers of the arterial wall. Blood leaks out, but is contained by the surrounding structures, creating a pulsatile hematoma.

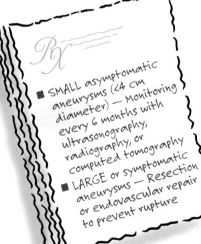

Rx

- SMALL asymptomatic aneurysms (<4 cm diameter) — Monitoring every 6 months with ultrasonography, radiography, or computed tomography
- LARGE or symptomatic aneurysms — Resection or endovascular repair to prevent rupture

Arterial occlusive disease

Arterial occlusive disease is a common complication of atherosclerosis. Obstruction or narrowing of the lumen of the aorta and its major branches causes an interruption of blood flow, usually to the legs and feet. It may affect the carotid, vertebral, subclavian, mesenteric, and celiac arteries and may be acute or chronic. Risk factors for arterial occlusive disease include smoking, aging, hypertension, hyperlipidemia, diabetes mellitus, and family history of vascular disorders, MI, or stroke. Men suffer from arterial occlusive disease more often than do women.

Arterial occlusive disease sites

- Vertebral
- Carotid
- Subclavian
- Celiac trunk
- Brachial
- Superior mesenteric trunk
- Inferior mesenteric
- Abdominal aorta
- Iliac
- Ulnar
- Radial
- Common femoral
- Superficial femoral
- Popliteal
- Posterior tibial
- Dorsalis pedis

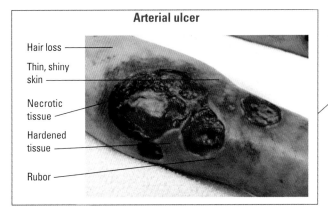

Arterial ulcer

- Hair loss
- Thin, shiny skin
- Necrotic tissue
- Hardened tissue
- Rubor

The five P's of acute occlusion

Pain

Pallor

Pulselessness

Paresthesia

Paralysis

memory board

Assessing peripheral arterial disease is easy. Remember that signs and symptoms may come in **PATCHES**:

Pulselessness

Altered appearance of affected extremity

Temperature differences

Capillary refill delay

Hardness of the tissue

Edema (minimal)

Sensation abnormalities (pain, tingling, numbness).

Treating arterial occlusive disease

Sir, I'm afraid we're looking at an occlusion here. I've got to ask you to stop smoking and clear the area.

All right, we're going to need to bring in the antiplatelet drugs and thrombolytic therapy to try to clear this backup.

If drugs don't work, invasive endovascular techniques, such as balloon angioplasty, atherectomy, and stenting, may be effective.

But if the obstruction still won't clear, a surgical intervention may be necessary.

Thrombophlebitis

Thrombophlebitis is an acute condition characterized by inflammation and thrombus formation in the veins. Alteration in the epithelial lining causes platelet aggregation and fibrin entrapment of red blood cells (RBCs), white blood cells, and additional platelets. The thrombus initiates a chemical inflammatory process in the vessel epithelium that leads to fibrosis, which may occlude the vessel lumen or embolize.

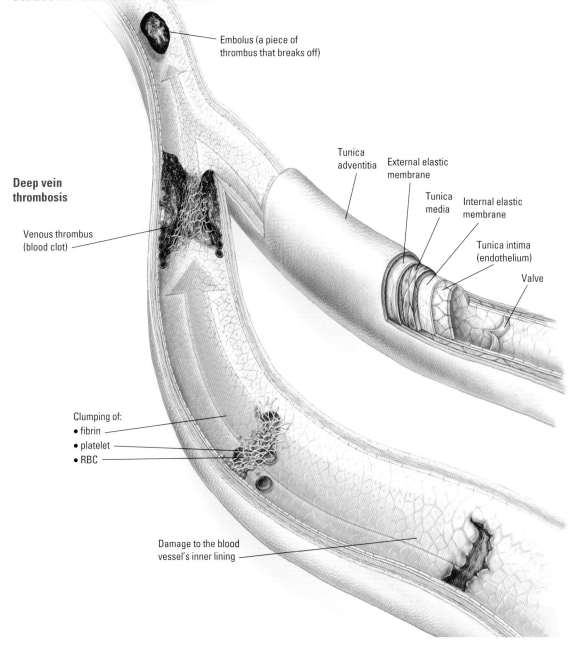

Embolus (a piece of thrombus that breaks off)

Tunica adventitia

External elastic membrane

Tunica media

Internal elastic membrane

Tunica intima (endothelium)

Valve

Deep vein thrombosis

Venous thrombus (blood clot)

Clumping of:
- fibrin
- platelet
- RBC

Damage to the blood vessel's inner lining

Superficial (subcutaneous) thrombophlebitis is usually self-limiting and rarely leads to pulmonary embolism.

Deep vein (intermuscular or intramuscular) thrombophlebitis can affect small veins as well as large veins, such as the vena cava and the femoral, iliac, and subclavian veins. Usually progressive, this disorder may lead to pulmonary embolism, a potentially fatal condition.

Signs and symptoms of superficial thrombophlebitis

Along the length of the affected vein:

- Heat
- Pain and tenderness
- Swelling
- Redness and induration

Signs and symptoms of DVT

- Fever and chills
- Malaise
- Severe pain and tenderness
- Swelling of the affected extremity
- Cyanosis of the extremity distal to the blockage
- Positive Homans' sign (although research has proven that this sign is not very reliable because it is not sensitive or specific to a DVT diagnosis) (Ambesh, Obiagwu, & Shetty, 2017)

Rx
- Bed rest with active and passive leg exercises
- Extremity elevation
- Analgesics, as needed
- Anticoagulants
- Graduated compression stockings

A patient with a high risk of thrombophlebitis and pulmonary embolus who also has contraindications to anticoagulant therapy or a high risk of bleeding might undergo insertion of a vena cava umbrella or filter.

My word!

Use the clues to help you unscramble the names of three common cardiovascular disorders. Then use the circled letters to answer the question posed.

Question: Which form of hypertension, also known as *primary hypertension*, is the most common type?

1. Diffuse inflammation of the cardiac muscle mytacosridi

— — — — ◯ — — — ◯ — ◯

2. Ineffective myocardial pumping hrate irefaul

— ◯ — — — — — ◯ — — —

3. Outpouching of the arterial wall actori mayersun

— — — — ◯ — — ◯◯ — — — ◯ —

Answer: ___ ___ ___ ___ ___ ___ ___ ___ ___ ___

Matchmaker

Match the three types of aneurysms shown here with their names.

1. _____   2. _____   3. _____

A. Saccular aortic

B. Fusiform

C. False

Selected References

Ambesh, P., Obiagwu, C., & Shetty, V. Homan's Sign for Deep Vein Thrombosis: A Grain of Salt? *Indian Heart Journal* 69(3):418–419, 2017.

Baddour, L.M., Wilson, W.R., Bayer, A.S., Fowler, V.G., Jr., Tleyjeh, I.M., Rybak, M.J., … Stroke Council. Infective Endocarditis in Adults: Diagnosis, Antimicrobial Therapy, and Management of Complications: A Scientific Statement for Healthcare Professionals from the American Heart Association, *Circulation* 132(15):1435–1486, 2015. doi:10.1161/CIR.0000000000000296

Domino, F.J. ed. *5-Minute Clinical Consult*, 25th ed. Philadelphia: Lippincott Williams & Wilkins Health, 2017.

Fihn, S.D., Blankenship, J.C., Alexander, K.P., Bittl, J.A., Byrne, J.G., Fletcher, B.J., … Society of Thoracic Surgeons. 2014 ACC/AHA/AATS/PCNA/SCAI/STS Focused Update of the Guideline for the Diagnosis and Management of Patients with Stable Ischemic Heart Disease: A Report of the American College of Cardiology/American Heart Association Task Force on Practice Guidelines, and the American Association for Thoracic Surgery, Preventive Cardiovascular Nurses Association, Society for Cardiovascular Angiography and Interventions, and Society of Thoracic Surgeons, *Journal of Thoracic and Cardiovascular Surgery* 149(3):e5-23, 2015. doi:10.1016/j.jtcvs.2014.11.002

Gerhard-Herman, M.D., Gornik, H.L., Barrett, C., Barshes, N.R., Corriere, M.A., Drachman, D.E., … Walsh, M.E. 2016 AHA/ACC Guideline on the Management of Patients with Lower Extremity Peripheral Artery Disease: A Report of the American College of Cardiology/American Heart Association Task Force on Clinical Practice Guidelines, *Circulation* 135(12):e726–e779, 2017. doi:10.1161/CIR.0000000000000471

Gersh, B.J., Maron, B.J., Bonow, R.O., Dearani, J.A., Fifer, M.A., Link, M.S., … Society of Thoracic Surgeons. 2011 ACCF/AHA Guideline for the Diagnosis and Treatment of Hypertrophic Cardiomyopathy: Executive Summary: A Report of the American College of Cardiology Foundation/American Heart Association Task Force on Practice Guidelines. *Circulation* 124(24):2761–2796, 2011. doi:10.1161/CIR.0b013e318223e230

Hiratzka, L.F., Bakris, G.L., Beckman, J.A., Bersin, R.M., Carr, V.F., Casey, D.E., Jr., … Society for Vascular Medicine. 2010 ACCF/AHA/AATS/ACR/ASA/SCA/SCAI/SIR/STS/SVM Guidelines for the Diagnosis and Management of Patients with Thoracic Aortic Disease: A Report of the American College of Cardiology Foundation/American Heart Association Task Force on Practice Guidelines, American Association for Thoracic Surgery, American College of Radiology, American Stroke Association, Society of Cardiovascular Anesthesiologists, Society for Cardiovascular Angiography and Interventions, Society of Interventional Radiology, Society of Thoracic Surgeons, and Society for Vascular Medicine, *Circulation* 121(13):e266–369, 2010. doi:10.1161/CIR.0b013e3181d4739e

James, P.A., Oparil, S., Carter, B.L., Cushman, W.C., Dennison-Himmelfarb, C., Handler, J., ... Ortiz, E. 2014 Evidence-Based Guideline for the Management of High Blood Pressure in Adults: Report from the Panel Members Appointed to the Eighth Joint National Committee (JNC 8), *JAMA* 311(5):507–520, 2014. doi:10.1001/jama.2013.284427

Kearon, C., Akl, E.A., Ornelas, J., Blaivas, A., Jimenez, D., Bounameaux, H., ... Moores, L. Antithrombotic Therapy for VTE Disease: CHEST Guideline and Expert Panel Report, *Chest* 149(2):315–352, 2016. doi:10.1016/j.chest.2015.11.026

Kindermann, I., Barth, C., Mahfoud, F., Ukena, C., Lenski, M., Yilmaz, A., ... Bohm, M. Update on Myocarditis, *J Am Coll Cardiol* 59(9):779–792, 2012. doi:10.1016/j.jacc.2011.09.074

Kumar, V., Abbas, A.K., Aster, J.C., & Perkins, J.A. *Robbins Basic Pathology*, 10th ed. Philadelphia: Elsevier, 2017.

Lilly, L.S. Treatment of Acute and Recurrent Idiopathic Pericarditis, *Circulation* 127(16):1723–1726, 2013. doi:10.1161/CIRCULATIONAHA.111.066365

Mann, D.L., Zipes, D.P., Libby, P., Bonow, R.O., & Braunwald, E. *Braunwald's Heart Disease: A Textbook of Cardiovascular Medicine*, 10th ed. Philadelphia: Elsevier/Saunders, 2015.

Nishimura, R.A., Otto, C.M., Bonow, R.O., Carabello, B.A., Erwin, J.P., III, Fleisher, L.A., ... Thompson, A. 2017 AHA/ACC Focused Update of the 2014 AHA/ACC Guideline for the Management of Patients with Valvular Heart Disease: A Report of the American College of Cardiology/American Heart Association Task Force on Clinical Practice Guidelines, *Circulation* 2017. doi:10.1161/CIR.0000000000000503

Nishimura, R.A., Otto, C.M., Bonow, R.O., Carabello, B.A., Erwin, J.P., III Guyton, R.A., ... American College of Cardiology/American Heart Association Task Force on Practice, Guidelines. 2014 AHA/ACC Guideline for the Management of Patients with Valvular Heart Disease: Executive Summary: A Report of the American College of Cardiology/American Heart Association Task Force on Practice Guidelines, *J Am Coll Cardiol* 63(22):2438–2488, 2014. doi:10.1016/j.jacc.2014.02.537

O'Gara, P.T., Kushner, F.G., Ascheim, D.D., Casey, D.E., Jr., Chung, M.K., de Lemos, J.A., ... American College of Cardiology Foundation/American Heart Association Task Force on Practice Guidelines. 2013 ACCF/AHA Guideline for the Management of ST-elevation Myocardial Infarction: A Report of the American College of Cardiology Foundation/American Heart Association Task Force on Practice Guidelines, *Circulation* 127(4):e362–425, 2013. doi:10.1161/CIR.0b013e3182742cf6

Taichman, D.B., Ornelas, J., Chung, L., Klinger, J.R., Lewis, S., Mandel, J., ... Badesch, D.B. Pharmacologic Therapy for Pulmonary Arterial Hypertension in Adults: CHEST Guideline and Expert Panel Report, *Chest* 146(2):449–475, 2014. doi:10.1378/chest.14-0793

Warnes, C.A., Williams, R.G., Bashore, T.M., Child, J.S., Connolly, H.M., Dearani, J.A., ... Webb, G.D. ACC/AHA 2008 Guidelines for the Management of Adults with Congenital Heart Disease: A Report of the American College of Cardiology/American Heart Association Task Force on Practice Guidelines (Writing Committee to Develop Guidelines on the Management of Adults with Congenital Heart Disease), *Circulation* 118(23):e714–833, 2008. doi:10.1161/CIRCULATIONAHA.108.190690

Yancy, C.W., Jessup, M., Bozkurt, B., Butler, J., Casey, D.E., Jr., Colvin, M.M., … Westlake, C. 2017 ACC/AHA/HFSA Focused Update of the 2013 ACCF/AHA Guideline for the Management of Heart Failure: A Report of the American College of Cardiology/American Heart Association Task Force on Clinical Practice Guidelines and the Heart Failure Society of America, *Circulation* 2017. doi:10.1161/CIR.0000000000000509

Chapter 7

Complications

Cardiogenic shock

Cardiogenic shock is a commonly fatal complication of various acute and chronic disorders that can cause cardiac decompensation. It can result from any condition that causes significant left ventricular dysfunction. Cardiac output is reduced, although vascular volume is adequate. The reduced cardiac output induces vasoconstriction that further reduces cardiac output and tissue perfusion. The reduced tissue perfusion leads to anaerobic metabolism and lactic acidosis. Acute myocardial infarction (MI) is the most common cause of cardiogenic shock. Other common causes of cardiogenic shock include valve stenosis, valve regurgitation, and cardiomyopathy.

Cardiogenic shock is sometimes called pump failure. It causes cardiac output to diminish, which severely impairs tissue perfusion.

Signs and symptoms

- Cyanosis
- Crackles
- Metabolic acidosis
- Cool, pale, clammy skin
- Weak, thready pulse
- Altered mentation

INCREASED

- Heart rate
- Respiratory rate
- Pulmonary artery pressure (PAP) and pulmonary artery wedge pressure (PAWP)
- B-type natriuretic peptide (BNP)
- Lactate

DECREASED

- Systolic pressure (<80 mm Hg)
- Urine output (<20 ml/hr)
- Pulse pressure
- Cardiac index
- Oxygen saturation

Cycle of decompensation

After an MI, even a slight reduction in cardiac output and arterial pressure can initiate a cycle of cardiac deterioration resulting in cardiogenic shock.

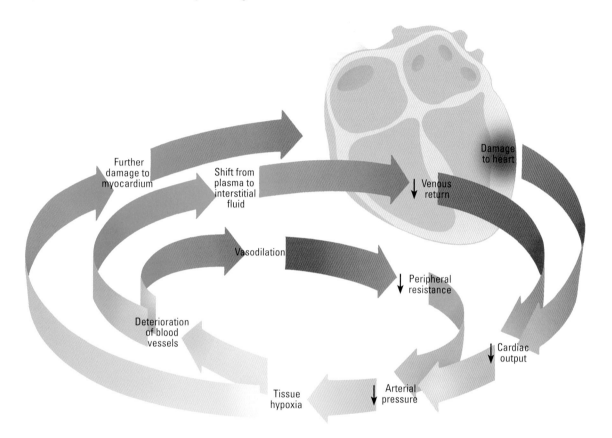

Further damage to myocardium

Shift from plasma to interstitial fluid

Damage to heart

↓ Venous return

Vasodilation

↓ Peripheral resistance

Deterioration of blood vessels

↓ Cardiac output

Tissue hypoxia

↓ Arterial pressure

Hemodynamic abnormalities in cardiogenic shock

Parameter	Abnormal value
Right atrial pressure	6 to 10 mm Hg
Right ventricular pressure	40 to 50/6 to 15 mm Hg
PAP	50/25 to 30 mm Hg
PAWP	25 to 40 mm Hg
Cardiac output	<4 L/min
Cardiac index	<2.5 L/min/m^2
Systemic vascular resistance	>2,000 dynes/sec/cm^{-5}

When drug therapy and an intra-aortic balloon pump (IABP) aren't enough, a ventricular assist device (VAD) may provide the next line of defense.

memory board

To help you recall the treatment protocol for cardiogenic shock, remember your ABCs (plus a D and an E).

Airway control with possible mechanical assistance

Breathing with high-flow rate oxygen therapy

Circulation monitoring and maintenance of large-bore intravenous (I.V.) lines

Drugs to increase cardiac output and stabilize the patient hemodynamically

Emergency IABP, VAD, or surgery

Rx

- Vasopressor agents, such as dopamine (Intropin), phenylephrine (Neo-Synephrine), or norepinephrine (Levophed)
- Inotropic agents, such as inamrinone (Amrinone) or dobutamine (Dobutrex)
- Nitrates, such as nitroglycerin (Tridil)
- Intra-aortic balloon pump (IABP) or left ventricular assist device (LVAD)
- Thrombolytic therapy or coronary artery revascularization
- Emergency surgery, if applicable

Hypovolemic shock

In hypovolemic shock, a reduction in intravascular volume causes circulatory dysfunction and inadequate tissue perfusion. This loss of volume results in a decrease in venous return to the right atrium, which then causes a decrease in cardiac output. Hypovolemic shock can be caused by acute blood or fluid loss — about 20% of total volume — that can result from:

- GI bleeding, internal or external hemorrhage, or any condition that reduces circulating intravascular volume or levels of other body fluids
- Dehydration from excessive perspiration, severe diarrhea, protracted vomiting, diabetes insipidus, diuresis, or inadequate fluid intake

Between a rock and a hard space

Third-space fluid shift can also cause hypovolemic shock. It can occur in the abdominal cavity (ascites), pleural cavity, or pericardial sac. Third spacing of fluid may occur in conditions such as intestinal obstruction, peritonitis, acute pancreatitis, and burns.

How hypovolemic shock occurs

The body initially tries to compensate for fluid loss; however, without prompt treatment, the body's compensatory mechanisms can't maintain circulation for long. Blood pressure falls dramatically and tissue perfusion decreases. The specific signs and symptoms that your patient exhibits will depend on the amount of fluid loss. Keep an eye out for these potential situations:

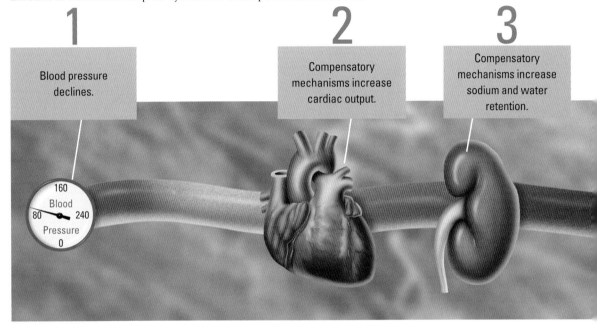

1 Blood pressure declines.

2 Compensatory mechanisms increase cardiac output.

3 Compensatory mechanisms increase sodium and water retention.

Estimating fluid loss

Changes in your patient's blood pressure, pulse rate, urine output, mental status, and skin condition signal whether fluid loss is minimal, moderate, or severe.

Key:
= Minimal fluid loss
= Moderate fluid loss
= Severe fluid loss

Your assessment findings will help you estimate the amount of fluid your patient has lost.

Blood pressure (mm Hg)

120
90
60

Supine systolic blood pressure

Pulse rate (beats/min)

160+
130
110

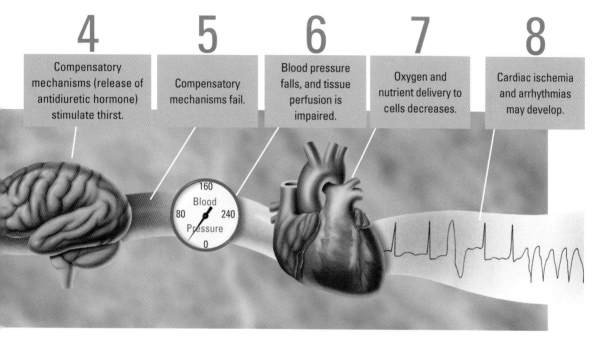

4 Compensatory mechanisms (release of antidiuretic hormone) stimulate thirst.

5 Compensatory mechanisms fail.

6 Blood pressure falls, and tissue perfusion is impaired.

7 Oxygen and nutrient delivery to cells decreases.

8 Cardiac ischemia and arrhythmias may develop.

160
Blood
80   240
Pressure
0

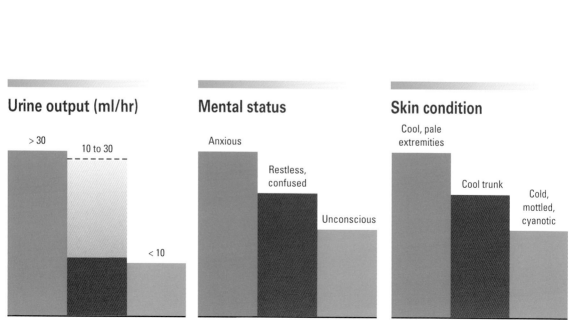

Urine output (ml/hr)

> 30

10 to 30

< 10

Mental status

Anxious

Restless, confused

Unconscious

Skin condition

Cool, pale extremities

Cool trunk

Cold, mottled, cyanotic

Signs and symptoms

- Cyanosis
- Metabolic acidosis
- Cool, pale, clammy skin
- Weak, thready pulse
- Orthostatic hypotension

INCREASED

- Heart rate
- Respiratory rate
- Urine specific gravity
- Lactate, creatinine, and blood urea nitrogen levels

DECREASED

- Sensorium
- Pulse pressure
- Urine output (less than 25 ml/hr)
- Blood pressure
- Central venous pressure (CVP), PAP, PAWP, and cardiac output
- Hemoglobin level and hematocrit (if hypovolemia is due to blood loss)

Positioning for shock

For years, patients in hypovolemic shock were placed in Trendelenburg's position. However, research now shows that only the legs should be elevated to avoid affecting gas exchange in the lungs or increasing intracranial pressure.

Cardiac tamponade

Cardiac tamponade is an unchecked increase in pressure in the pericardium or pericardial sac. It results from blood or fluid that accumulates in the sac and compresses the heart. This compression obstructs blood flow into the ventricles and reduces the amount of blood pumped out of the heart with each contraction. Possible causes include Dressler's syndrome, MI, pericarditis, malignant effusions, blunt or penetrating precordial trauma, or collagen diseases such as lupus.

MI and cardiac tamponade

A ruptured, cardiac muscle (as a result of an MI) causes a massive accumulation of blood in the pericardial cavity. The result is cardiac tamponade.

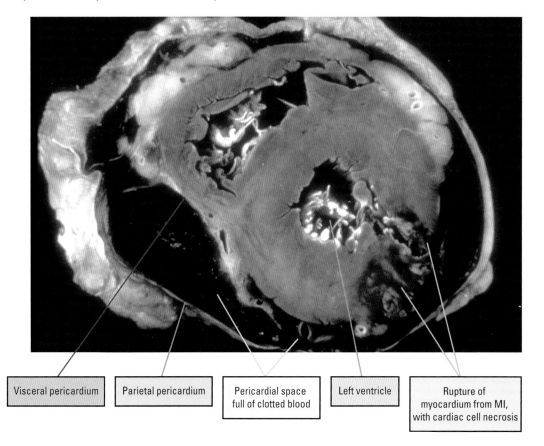

Visceral pericardium

Parietal pericardium

Pericardial space full of clotted blood

Left ventricle

Rupture of myocardium from MI, with cardiac cell necrosis

Understanding cardiac tamponade

Normal heart and pericardium

The pericardial space normally contains 10 to 30 ml of pericardial fluid, which lubricates the layers of the heart and reduces friction when the heart contracts.

Aorta

Superior vena cava

Fibrous pericardium

Parietal pericardium

Visceral pericardium

Pericardial space

Attachment of fibrous pericardium to diaphragm

Diaphragm

Cardiac tamponade

In cardiac tamponade, blood or fluid fills the pericardial space, compressing the heart, decreasing cardiac output, and obstructing venous return.

Even a small amount of fluid — 50 to 100 ml — can be fatal if it accumulates rapidly.

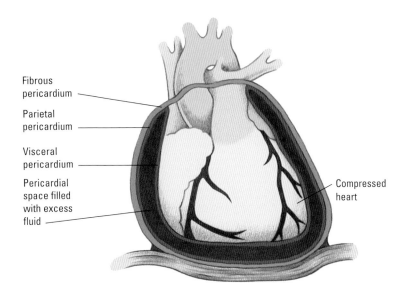

Fibrous pericardium

Parietal pericardium

Visceral pericardium

Pericardial space filled with excess fluid

Compressed heart

Signs and symptoms

The three classic signs of cardiac tamponade (Beck's triad) are:
- elevated CVP with jugular vein distention
- muffled heart sounds
- pulsus paradoxus (inspiratory drop in systemic blood pressure greater than 15 mm Hg).

Other signs and symptoms include:
- hypotension
- tachycardia
- weak, thready pulses
- chest pain
- restlessness or anxiety
- CVP = PAWP
- decreased cardiac output

Cardiac tamponade has three classic features known as Beck's triad.

Understanding signs and symptoms of cardiac tamponade

Syncope, anxiety, and restlessness due to decreased oxygenation

Jugular vein distention due to elevated CVP

Dyspnea and cough due to compressed trachea and bronchi

Decreased vital capacity

Pulsus paradoxus due to arterial compression during inhalation

Muffled heart sounds due to fluid accumulation

Compression of the heart due to pressure from the pericardial sac

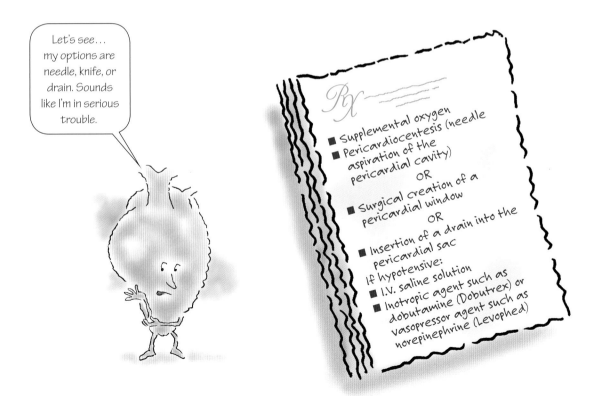

Myocardial contusion

A myocardial contusion (bruising of the myocardium) is the most common type of injury sustained from blunt trauma, such as a fall or impact from a steering wheel or other object. The right ventricle is the most common site of injury because of its location directly behind the sternum.

With deceleration injuries, the myocardium may strike the sternum and become injured. In addition, the aorta may be lacerated from shear force. Direct force applied to the sternum can also cause myocardium contusion.

Signs and symptoms

- Arrhythmias
- Contusions on the chest
- Precordial chest pain
- Dyspnea
- Pericardial friction rub
- Hemodynamic instability
- Cardiac tamponade
- Tachycardia

℞
- Supplemental oxygen
- Analgesic medications
- I.V. fluid therapy
If contusion causes hemodynamic instability, other medications may be needed:
- Antiarrhythmics
- Digoxin
- Inotropic agents

Sternum

Right ventricle

Pseudoaneurysm

A pseudoaneurysm forms when trauma to the arterial wall causes blood to leak into surrounding tissues, forming a pulsatile hematoma. Pseudoaneurysms are commonly caused by interventional or catheterization procedures in which large catheters and sheaths are used to cannulate arteries. They're also a common complication from vascular surgery. Less commonly, they may be caused by an infection or cancer that damages the arterial wall.

Signs and symptoms

- Swelling and pain at insertion site
- Pulsatile mass
- Bruit
- Palpable thrill
- "To and fro" murmur over mass
- Extensive ecchymosis

> Small pseudoaneurysms may spontaneously thrombose and not require treatment.

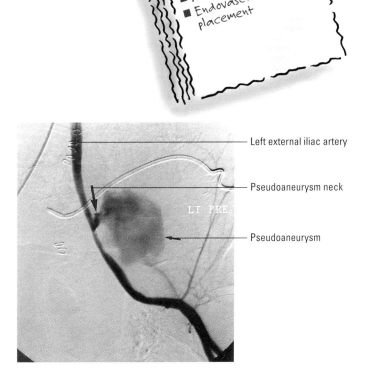

Rx
- Ultrasound-guided direct compression maneuvers
- Thrombin injection
- Arterioplasty
- Endovascular stent placement

Left external iliac artery

Pseudoaneurysm neck

LT PRE

Pseudoaneurysm

Pericarditis

Pericarditis is an inflammation of the membranous sac around the heart. The inflammatory process causes an increase in the amount of fluid in the pericardial sac. If unchecked, this accumulation could cause cardiac tamponade. Pericarditis can develop as a consequence of infectious or noninfectious causes such as MI or uremia.

Signs and Symptoms
- Chest pain (Tip: the chest pain of pericarditis is sharp and can be relieved by sitting up and leaning forward)
- Pericardial friction rub
- Tachycardia
- Tachypnea
- Fever
- ECG changes

Treatment
- Nonsteroidal anti-inflammatory drugs (NSAIDs), such as ibuprofen (Motrin) or indomethacin (Indocin)
- Antibiotics (if infectious in nature)
- Hemodialysis (if uremic in nature)

Rebus riddle

Sound out each group of symbols and letters to reveal a fact about a cardiovascular complication.

My word!

Unscramble the names of four terms related to cardiac tamponade. Then, use the circled letters to answer the question posed.

Question: What name is given to the three classic signs of cardiac tamponade?

1. carriedpail capes

— — — — — ◯ — — ◯ — —   ◯ —

— — —

2. mrspoonsice

◯ — — — ◯ — — — — — — —

3. lobdo tunicacoalum

◯ — — — — — — — — — — — —

— — ◯ — — —

4. needchuck canesire

___ ___ ___ ___ ___ ___ ⃝ ___ ⃝ ___ ___ ___

___ ___ ⃝ ___ ___

Answer: ___ ___ ___ ___'___ ___ ___ ___ ___

Answers: Rebus riddle Cardiogenic shock is sometimes called pump failure. My word! 1. Pericardial space, 2. Compression, 3. Blood accumulation, 4. Unchecked increase; Question: Beck's triad

---

Suggested references

Annane, D., Siami, S., Jaber, S., Martin, C., Elatrous, S., Declere, A.D., … Chevret, S. Effects of Fluid Resuscitation with Colloids Vs Crystalloids on Mortality in Critically Ill Patients Presenting with Hypovolemic Shock: The CRISTAL Randomized Trial. *Journal of the American Medical Association* 10(17): 1809–1817, 2013.

Bhat, T., Teli, S., Bhat, H., Akhtar, M., Meghani, M., Lafferty, J., & Gala, B. Access-Site Complications and Their Management during Transradial Cardiac Catheterization. *Expert Review of Cardiovascular Therapy* 10(5):627–634, 2012. doi:http://dx.doi.org/10.1586/erc.12.16

Cabrera, G., & Schub, T. *Pericarditis.* 2015. Retrieved *Cinahl Nursing Guide* from: http://ezproxy.harford.edu/login?url=http://search.ebscohost.com/login.aspx?direct=true&db=nrc&AN=T701154&site=nrc-live

Cooper, H.A., & Panza, J.A. Cardiogenic Shock. *Cardiology Clinics* 31(4):567–580, 2013. doi:10.1016/j.ccl.2013.07.009

Curry, S. Acute Pericarditis: An Overview. *British Journal of Cardiac Nursing* 9(3): 124–131, 2014. doi:10.12968/bjca.2014.9.3.124

Ergle, K., Parto, P., & Krim, S.R. Percutaneous Ventricular Assist Devices: A Novel Approach in the Management of Patients with Acute Cardiogenic Shock. *The Ochsner Journal* 16(3):243–249, 2016. Retrieved from http://ezproxy.harford.edu/login?url=https://search.proquest.com/docview/1820582888?accountid=11292

Hoffmann, J., & Sullivan, N., eds. *Medical-Surgical Nursing: Making Connections to Practice.* Philadelphia, PA: F.A. Davis, 2017.

Hollenberg, S.M. Vasoactive Drugs in Circulatory Shock. *American Journal of Respiratory and Critical Care Medicine* 183(7):847–855, 2011. Retrieved from http://ezproxy.harford.edu/login?url=https://search.proquest.com/docview/860038671?accountid=1129

Imazio, M. Evaluation and Management of Pericarditis. *Expert Review of Cardiovascular Therapy* 9(9):1221–1233, 2011. doi:http://dx.doi.org/10.1586/erc.11.111 11292

Imazio, M., & Adler, Y. Management of Pericardial Effusion. *European Heart Journal* 34(16):1186–1197, 2013. doi:10.1093/eurheartj/ehs372

Joos, E., Tadloc, M.D., & Inaba, K. Diagnosis, Work-Up and Management of Blunt Cardiac Injuries. *Trauma* 16(2):93–98, 2014. doi:http://dx.doi.org/10.1177/1460408614525740

Khandaker, M.H., Espinosa, R.E., Nishimura, R.A., Sinak, L.J., Hayes, S.N., Melduni, R.M., & Oh, J.K. Pericardial Disease: Diagnosis and Management. *Mayo Clinic Proceedings* 85(6):572–593, 2010. Retrieved from http://ezproxy.harford.edu/login?url=https://search.proquest.com/docview/366562601?accountid=11292

Kolecki, P. *Hypovolemic Shock Treatment & Management*. 2014. Retrieved from http://emedicine.medscape.com/article/760145-treatment

Levy, B., Bastien, O., Karim, B., Cariou, A., Chouihed, T., Combes, A., … Kuteifan, K. (2015). Experts' Recommendations for the Management of Adult Patients with Cardiogenic Shock. *Annals of Intensive Care* 5(1):1–10. doi:http://dx.doi.org/10.1186/s13613-015-0052-1

Lewis, S., Bucher, L., Heitkemper, M., & Harding, M., eds. *Medical-Surgical Nursing: Assessment and Management of Clinical Problems*, 10th ed. St. Louis, MO: Elsevier, 2017.

Schub, T., & Boling, B. *Cardiac Tamponade*. 2013. Retrieved *Cinahl Nursing Guide* from http://ezproxy.harford.edu/login?url=http://search.ebscohost.com/login.aspx?direct=true&db=nrc&AN=T701199&site=nrc-live

Schub, T., & March, P. *Shock, Hypovolemic*. 2014. Retrieved *Cinahl Nursing Guide* from http://ezproxy.harford.edu/login?url=http://search.ebscohost.com/login.aspx?direct=true&db=nrc&AN=T701249&site=nrc-live

Schub, T., March, P., & Pravikoff, D. *Shock, Cardiogenic*. 2016. Retrieved *Cinahl Nursing Guide* from http://ezproxy.harford.edu/login?url=http://search.ebscohost.com/login.aspx?direct=true&db=nrc&AN=T701253&site=nrc-live

Solomon, C.G., & LeWinter, M.M. Acute Pericarditis. *The New England Journal of Medicine* 371(25):2410–2416, 2014. Retrieved from http://ezproxy.harford.edu/login?url=https://search.proquest.com/docview/1638897591?accountid=11292

Chapter 8

Treatments

Drug therapy

As far as class I antiarrhythmics go, I'm a class act, but I'm also in a class of my own.

Antiarrhythmics

Antiarrhythmics are used to treat disturbances in normal heart rhythm and are grouped in one of four classes.

Drugs are an important part of treatment for cardiac disorders.

Class	Features	Rhythms treated	Examples
I Sodium channel blockers	♥ Largest class ♥ Three subdivisions plus adenosine ♥ Decrease automaticity, conduction velocity, and membrane responsiveness	♥ IA: atrial and ventricular arrhythmias ♥ IB: acute ventricular arrhythmias ♥ IC: severe refractory ventricular arrhythmias ♥ Adenosine: paroxysmal supraventricular tachycardia	♥ IA: disopyramide (Norpace) ♥ IB: lidocaine (Xylocaine) ♥ IC: flecainide (Tambocor)
II Beta-adrenergic blockers	♥ Slow automaticity of sinoatrial (SA) node ♥ Reduce conduction of atrioventricular (AV) node and pacer cells ♥ Decrease strength of contraction	♥ Atrial flutter and fibrillation ♥ Paroxysmal atrial tachycardia	♥ Atenolol (Tenormin) ♥ Metoprolol (Lopressor) ♥ Propranolol (Inderal) ♥ Carvedilol (Coreg) ♥ Nebivolol (Bystolic)
III Diverse group	♥ Mechanism of action poorly understood ♥ May slow repolarization ♥ May prolong refractory period	♥ Ventricular arrhythmias	♥ Amiodarone (Cordarone) ♥ Dofetilide (Tikosyn) ♥ Sotalol (Betapace) ♥ Ibutilide (Corvert)
IV Calcium channel blockers	♥ Decrease cardiac contractility and oxygen demand ♥ Dilate coronary arteries and arterioles	♥ Supraventricular arrhythmias with rapid ventricular response	♥ Diltiazem (Cardizem) ♥ Nifedipine (Procardia) ♥ Verapamil (Calan)

Inotropic drugs

Inotropics increase the force of the heart's contractions. There are two types:
- digoxin (Lanoxin), which slows the heart rate and electrical impulse conduction through the SA and AV nodes
- phosphodiesterase (PDE) inhibitors, which provide short-term management of heart failure or long-term management in patients awaiting heart transplant surgery. Two examples of PDE inhibitors are inamrinone and milrinone.

PDE inhibitors should be administered only via I.V.

Antianginals

Antianginals relieve chest pain (angina) by reducing myocardial oxygen demand, increasing the supply of oxygen to the heart, or both. There are three main types:
- nitrates (used primarily to treat acute angina)
- beta-adrenergic blockers (prescribed for long-term prevention of angina)
- Ranolazine (Ranexa) prescribed for patients with ischemic stable heart disease, if unable to tolerate acceptable doses of beta-blockers (Montalescot et al., 2013)
- calcium channel blockers (used when other drugs fail to prevent angina).

How antianginal drugs work

When the coronary arteries can't supply enough oxygen to the myocardium, angina occurs. This forces the heart to work harder, increasing heart rate, preload, afterload, and the force of myocardial contractility. Antianginal drugs relieve angina by decreasing one or more of these four factors.

Nitrates can be quick or slow acting. It all depends on the delivery route and the drug.

Afterload
- Calcium channel blockers
- Nitrates

Heart rate
- Beta-adrenergic blockers
- Calcium channel blockers

Preload
- Nitrates

Contractility
- Beta-adrenergic blockers
- Calcium channel blockers

Antihypertensives

Treatment for hypertension begins with modifying diet, encouraging exercise, and, if indicated, counseling about weight loss. If these measures aren't enough, drugs can help.

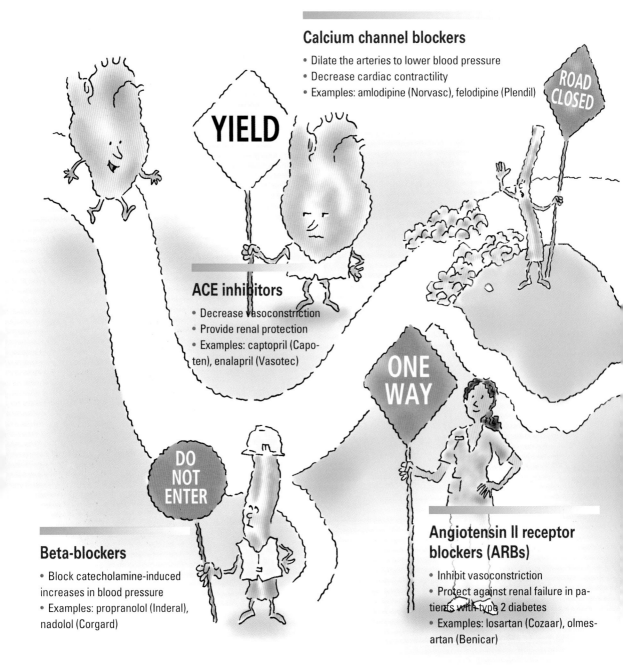

Calcium channel blockers
- Dilate the arteries to lower blood pressure
- Decrease cardiac contractility
- Examples: amlodipine (Norvasc), felodipine (Plendil)

ACE inhibitors
- Decrease vasoconstriction
- Provide renal protection
- Examples: captopril (Capoten), enalapril (Vasotec)

Beta-blockers
- Block catecholamine-induced increases in blood pressure
- Examples: propranolol (Inderal), nadolol (Corgard)

Angiotensin II receptor blockers (ARBs)
- Inhibit vasoconstriction
- Protect against renal failure in patients with type 2 diabetes
- Examples: losartan (Cozaar), olmesartan (Benicar)

Sympatholytics

* Decrease peripheral vascular resistance by inhibiting the sympathetic nervous system
* Examples: clonidine (Catapres), doxazosin (Cardura), carvedilol (Coreg)

Direct renin inhibitors

* Block renin and help blood vessels relax
* Example: aliskiren (Tekturna)

Diuretics

* Help kidneys excrete water and electrolytes, which lowers blood pressure
* Thiazide example: hydrochlorothiazide (HydroDIURIL)
* Loop example: furosemide (Lasix)
* Potassium sparing, example: triamterene (spironolactone) and Dyrenium (Aldactone) (http://www.mayoclinic.org/diseases-conditions/high-blood-pressure/in-depth/diuretics/art-20048129)

Selective aldosterone receptor antagonists

* Used as a second-line treatment when other drugs fail
* Eplerenone (Inspra), spironolactone (Aldactone) (https://www.drugs.com/drug-class/aldosterone-receptor-antagonists.html)

Vasodilators

* Relax arteries, veins, or both
* Oral example: hydralazine

For hypertensive crisis

* Example: I.V. nitroprusside (Nitropress)

Treating hypertension

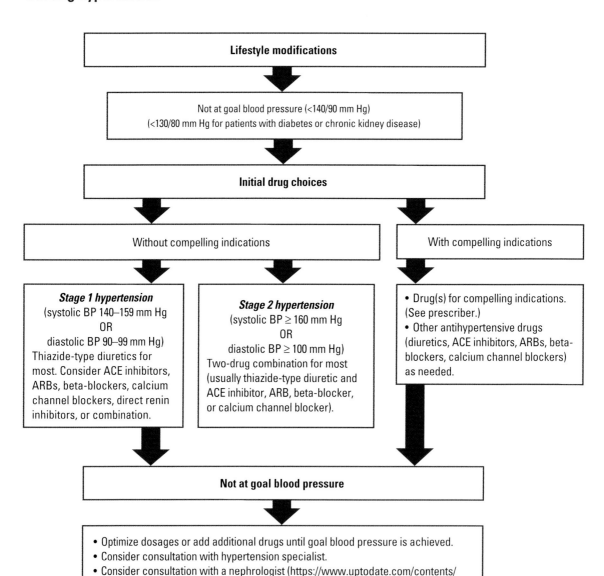

Lifestyle modifications

↓

Not at goal blood pressure (<140/90 mm Hg)
(<130/80 mm Hg for patients with diabetes or chronic kidney disease)

↓

Initial drug choices

Without compelling indications

With compelling indications

Stage 1 hypertension
(systolic BP 140–159 mm Hg
OR
diastolic BP 90–99 mm Hg)
Thiazide-type diuretics for
most. Consider ACE inhibitors,
ARBs, beta-blockers, calcium
channel blockers, direct renin
inhibitors, or combination.

Stage 2 hypertension
(systolic BP ≥ 160 mm Hg
OR
diastolic BP ≥ 100 mm Hg)
Two-drug combination for most
(usually thiazide-type diuretic and
ACE inhibitor, ARB, beta-blocker,
or calcium channel blocker).

• Drug(s) for compelling indications.
(See prescriber.)
• Other antihypertensive drugs
(diuretics, ACE inhibitors, ARBs, beta-
blockers, calcium channel blockers)
as needed.

Not at goal blood pressure

• Optimize dosages or add additional drugs until goal blood pressure is achieved.
• Consider consultation with hypertension specialist.
• Consider consultation with a nephrologist (https://www.uptodate.com/contents/
treatment-of-resistant-hypertension)

Antihypertensives and the RAAS

The renin-angiotensin-aldosterone system (RAAS) regulates the body's sodium and water levels and blood pressure.

1. Juxtaglomerular cells near the glomeruli in each kidney secrete the enzyme renin into the blood.

2. Renin circulates throughout the body and converts angiotensinogen, made in the liver, to angiotensin I.

3. In the lungs, angiotensin I is converted by hydrolysis to angiotensin II.

4. Angiotensin II acts on the adrenal cortex to stimulate production of the hormone aldosterone. Aldosterone acts on the juxtaglomerular cells to increase sodium and water retention and to stimulate or depress further renin secretion, completing the feedback system that automatically readjusts homeostasis.

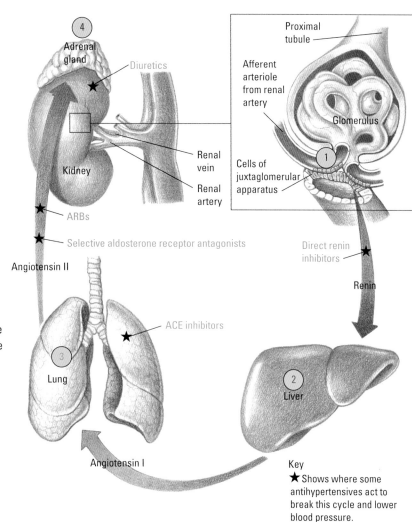

Key
★ Shows where some antihypertensives act to break this cycle and lower blood pressure.

Adverse reactions of antihypertensive drugs

All	ACE inhibitors	ARBs	Direct renin inhibitors
• Headache	• Altered renal function when used with nonsteroidal anti-inflammatory drugs	• Transient elevations of blood urea nitrogen and serum creatinine levels	• Dizziness
• Fatigue			• Fainting
• Angioedema			• Diarrhea
• GI reactions	• Dry, nonproductive, persistent cough	• Cough	
• Electrolyte imbalance (specific to drug used)		• Tickling in throat	

Antilipemics

Antilipemics lower cholesterol, triglyceride, and phospholipid levels. They're used in combination with lifestyle modification to decrease the risk of coronary artery disease (CAD).

To lower cholesterol levels, combine pharmacologic therapy with lifestyle modification.

Cholesterol absorption inhibitors

- Lower total cholesterol levels
- Example: ezetimibe (Zetia)

Nicotinic acid (niacin)

- Water-soluble vitamin
- Lowers triglyceride levels
- Increases high-density lipoprotein (HDL) levels
- Example: niacin (Niacor)

Bile-sequestering drugs

- Remove excess bile acids from fat deposits
- Lower low-density lipoprotein (LDL) levels
- Example: cholestyramine (Questran)

Fibric acid derivatives

- Lower triglyceride levels
- Minimally increase HDL levels
- Examples: fenofibrate (Tricor), gemfibrozil (Lopid)

HMG-CoA reductase inhibitors

- Also known as *statins*
- Lower total cholesterol and LDL levels
- Minimally increase HDL levels
- Examples: atorvastatin (Lipitor), simvastatin (Zocor), rosuvastatin (Crestor)

Anticoagulants

Anticoagulants reduce the blood's ability to clot. They're prescribed for mitral insufficiency or atrial fibrillation or to dissolve clots that block an artery.

Antiplatelets

Antiplatelets interfere with the binding of platelets or the process preceding the blood clotting process (http://www.healthline.com/health/anticoagulant-and-antiplatelet-drugs#overview16).

Category	Features	Examples
Heparins	♥ Used in patients with unstable angina, MI, and deep vein thrombosis (DVT) ♥ Acts immediately when given I.V. ♥ Available in regular and low molecular weight forms	♥ Heparin (Liquaemin) *Low molecular weight* ♥ Dalteparin (Fragmin) ♥ Enoxaparin (Lovenox)
Coumarin derivative	♥ Antagonizes production of vitamin K–dependent clotting factors ♥ Prevents DVT ♥ Used in patients who have undergone prosthetic heart valve surgery and those with diseased valves ♥ Given orally and takes days to reach effect	♥ Warfarin (Coumadin)
Antiplatelet drugs	♥ Prevent thromboembolism	♥ Brilinta (Ticagrelor) ♥ Clopidogrel (Plavix)
Direct thrombin inhibitors (IIa)	♥ Treat heparin-induced thrombocytopenia ♥ Used when heparin can't be ♥ Prophylactically used before angioplasty and stent placement ♥ Available I.V.	♥ Argatroban ♥ Bivalirudin (Angiomax) ♥ Lepirudin (Refludan)
Glycoprotein IIb/IIIa inhibitors	♥ Used in patients with unstable angina and before and during angioplasty ♥ Prevent platelets from binding together ♥ Available I.V.	♥ Abciximab (ReoPro) ♥ Eptifibatide (Integrilin) ♥ Tirofiban (Aggrastat)

Thrombolytics

Thrombolytics can dissolve a preexisting clot or thrombus in acute MI, ischemic stroke, or peripheral artery occlusion. They also can dissolve thrombi and reestablish blood flow in arteriovenous cannulas and I.V. catheters. In an acute or emergent situation, they must be administered within 3 to 6 hours after the onset of symptoms. Thrombolytics include alteplase (Activase), reteplase (Retavase), urokinase (Abbokinase), and tenecteplase (TNKase).

How thrombolytics help restore circulation

When a thrombus forms in an artery, it obstructs the blood supply, causing ischemia and necrosis. Thrombolytics can dissolve thrombi in the coronary and pulmonary arteries, restoring the blood supply to the area beyond the blockage.

Obstructed artery

A thrombus blocks blood flow through the artery, causing distal ischemia.

Blood supply

Thrombus

Ischemic area

Artery wall

Inside the thrombus

The thrombolytic enters the thrombus and binds to the fibrin-plasminogen complex, converting inactive plasminogen into active plasmin. Active plasmin digests fibrin, dissolving the thrombus. As the thrombus dissolves, blood flow resumes.

Thrombolytic

Plasminogen

Fibrin strand

Active plasmin

Break in fibrin strand

Treatments for CAD

Coronary artery bypass graft surgery

Coronary artery bypass graft (CABG) surgery relieves the symptoms of CAD and decreases risk of future heart attack or heart failure. Watch patients who have had CABG surgery for such complications as severe hypotension, decreased cardiac output, and cardiogenic shock.

Greater
saphenous
vein (donor vein) —

CABG circumvents an occluded coronary artery by using a segment of the saphenous vein, radial artery, or internal mammary artery to restore blood flow to the heart.

Greater saphenous
vein graft

Photo op

Performing CABG surgery

CABG surgery is performed either "on pump" (the traditional method) or "off pump" (also called the "beating heart method" or OPCAB). A technician monitors the heart-lung machine (cardiopulmonary bypass pump), shown below.

Donor
vein

Sutures

The road to recovery

Here are the landmarks that you'll want to look for on your patient's postoperative CABG road to recovery.

Minimally invasive direct coronary artery bypass

Minimally invasive direct coronary artery bypass (MIDCAB) is a less invasive surgical treatment for CAD. Because the procedure is minimally invasive, it results in shorter hospital stays, fewer postoperative complications, earlier extubation, reduced cost, smaller incisions, and an earlier return to work.

The MIDCAB procedure

MIDCAB is performed through several small incisions in the left chest cavity. The internal mammary artery is sewn to the left anterior descending artery in the front of the heart, as shown here. The patient receives only right lung ventilation and drugs to slow the heart rate and reduce heart movement during surgery.

> With MIDCAB, I'm back on my feet in no time.

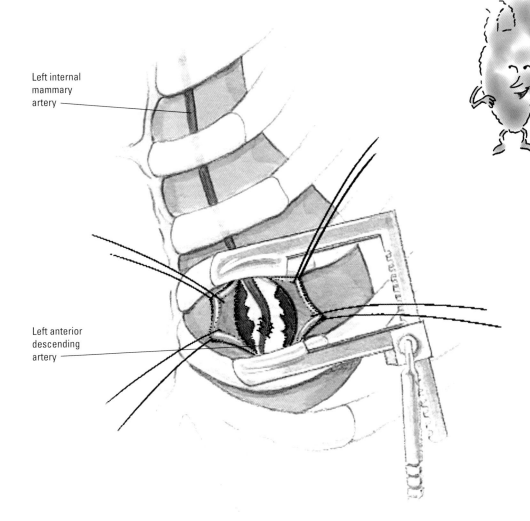

Left internal mammary artery

Left anterior descending artery

Comparing types of CABG

Features	On-pump CABG	OPCAB	MIDCAB
Access site	♥ Breastbone severed for heart access	♥ Breastbone severed for heart access	♥ Incisions made between ribs for anterior heart access, no bones cut
Indications	♥ Suitable for multivessel disease, any coronary artery	♥ Suitable for multivessel disease, any coronary artery	♥ Only used for one-vessel diseases in anterior portions of the heart, such as left anterior descending artery, or some portions of the right coronary and circumflex arteries
Graft types	♥ Combination of artery and vein grafts	♥ Combination of artery and vein grafts	♥ Arterial grafts (better long-term results)
Complications	♥ Highest risk of post-operative complications	♥ Reduced blood usage, fewer rhythm problems, less kidney dysfunction than on-pump CABG	♥ Reduced blood usage, fewest complications, fastest recovery
Intubation	♥ Up to 24 hours	♥ Up to 24 hours	♥ Usually for 2 to 4 hours
Incisions	♥ Leg incisions for vein grafting, possibly arm incision for radial artery grafting	♥ Leg incisions for vein grafting, possibly arm incision for radial artery grafting	♥ No leg incisions, possibly arm incision for radial artery grafting
Heart and lung function	♥ Heart and lung circulation bypassed mechanically, affecting blood cells	♥ Drugs and special equipment used to slow heart and immobilize it; cardiopulmonary and systemic circulation still function	♥ Drugs used to slow heart; cardiopulmonary and systemic circulation still function

Of the three types of CABG surgery, MIDCAB is the least invasive and has the fewest complications.

Percutaneous transluminal coronary angioplasty

Percutaneous transluminal coronary angioplasty (PTCA), also called *angioplasty*, is a nonsurgical alternative to CABG. Performed in the cardiac catheterization laboratory, under local anesthesia, it involves the use of a balloon-tipped catheter to dilate the blocked coronary artery. In most cases, patients recuperate quickly, usually walking the same day and returning to work in 2 weeks.

PTCA works best when lesions are readily accessible, noncalcified, less than 10 mm, concentric, discrete, and smoothly tapered. Possible complications include acute vessel closure and late restenosis.

Understanding PTCA

In PTCA, a guide catheter is threaded into the coronary artery. Then, a balloon-tipped catheter is inserted through the occlusion and inflated and deflated to flatten the plaque until the vessel is opened.

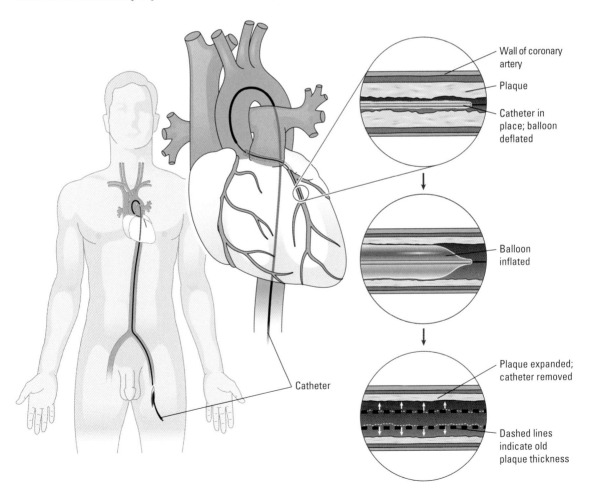

Intravascular stents

An intravascular stent may be used to hold the walls of a vessel open. Some stents are coated with a drug that's slowly released to inhibit further aggregation of fibrin or clots.

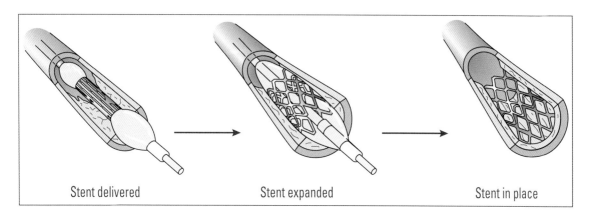

Stent delivered   Stent expanded   Stent in place

Atherectomy

Atherectomy is the use of a small, rotating knife to remove fatty deposits from blocked coronary arteries. The catheter is advanced to the arterial obstruction, the knife is positioned precisely on the fatty deposit, and then the fatty deposit is shaved off the artery wall.

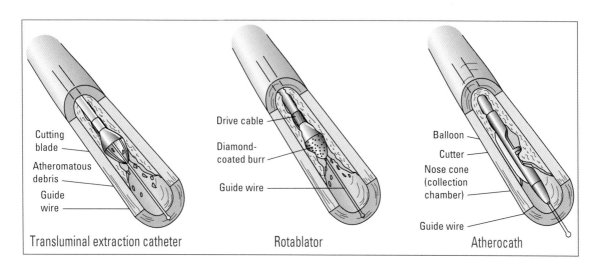

Transluminal extraction catheter   Rotablator   Atherocath

IABP counterpulsation

Intra-aortic balloon pump (IABP) counterpulsation temporarily reduces left ventricular workload and improves coronary perfusion. It's used to treat cardiogenic shock caused by acute MI, septic shock, intractable angina before surgery, intractable ventricular arrhythmias, ventricular septal or papillary muscle ruptures, and pump failure.

Understanding an IABP

An IABP consists of a polyurethane balloon attached to an external pump console by means of a large-lumen catheter. It's inserted percutaneously through the femoral artery and positioned in the descending aorta, just distal to the left subclavian artery and above the renal arteries.

Push

This external pump works in precise counterpoint to the left ventricle, inflating the balloon with helium early in diastole and deflating it just before systole. As the balloon inflates, it forces blood toward the aortic valve, thereby raising pressure in the aortic root and augmenting diastolic pressure to improve coronary perfusion. It also improves peripheral circulation by forcing blood through the brachiocephalic, common carotid, and subclavian arteries arising from the aortic trunk.

...and pull

The balloon deflates rapidly at the end of diastole, creating a vacuum in the aorta. This reduces aortic volume and pressure, thereby decreasing the resistance to left ventricular ejection (afterload). This decreased workload, in turn, reduces the heart's oxygen requirements and, combined with the improved myocardial perfusion, helps prevent or diminish myocardial ischemia.

Diastole

Systole

The balloon inflates during early diastole...

...AND DEFLATES JUST BEFORE SYSTOLE.

Timing IABP counterpulsation

IABP counterpulsation is synchronized with either the electrocardiogram or the arterial waveform. Ideally, balloon inflation should begin when the aortic valve closes — at the dicrotic notch on the arterial waveform. Deflation should occur just before systole.

When the time is right

Timing is crucial. Early inflation can damage the aortic valve by forcing it closed, whereas late inflation permits most of the blood emerging from the ventricle to flow past the balloon, reducing pump effectiveness.

Late deflation may cause cardiac arrest because it increases the resistance to left ventricle pumping.

At the peak

IABP counterpulsation boosts peak diastolic pressure and lowers peak systolic and end-diastolic pressures.

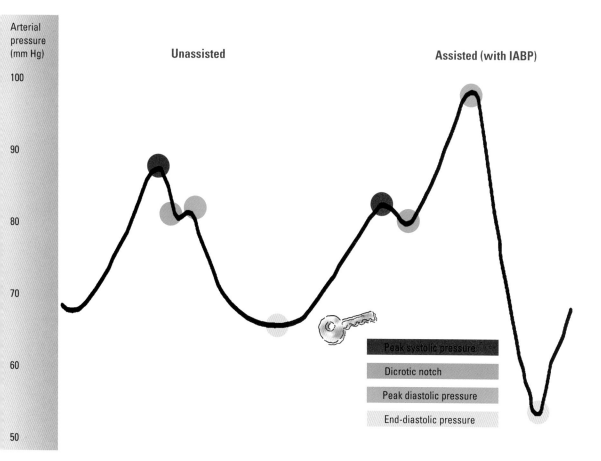

Enhanced external counterpulsation

Enhanced external counterpulsation (EECP) provides pain relief for patients who suffer from recurrent stable angina when standard treatments fail. It's a noninvasive technique that increases oxygen-rich blood flow to the heart and reduces the heart's workload. EECP can reduce angina pain, improve exercise tolerance, and stimulate collateral circulation.

EECP treatment

In EECP, three pneumatic cuffs are wrapped around the patient's calves, thighs, and lower buttocks. These cuffs are synchronized with the heart rate and sequentially inflate and gently compress blood vessels in the legs, forcing blood back to the heart.

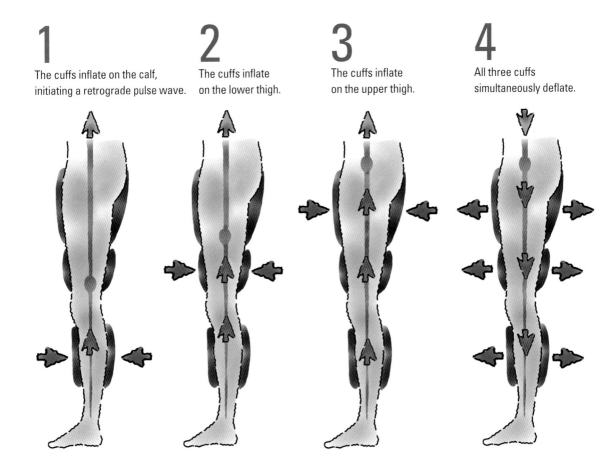

1 The cuffs inflate on the calf, initiating a retrograde pulse wave.

2 The cuffs inflate on the lower thigh.

3 The cuffs inflate on the upper thigh.

4 All three cuffs simultaneously deflate.

Cardiac rehabilitation

Cardiac rehabilitation is a medically supervised program, with a major objective of improving the cardiac health of those burdened with a history of heart attack, heart failure, angioplasty, or cardiac surgery (http://www.heart.org/ HEARTORG/Conditions/More/CardiacRehab/What-is-Cardiac-Rehabilitation_ UCM_307049_Article.jsp#.WQkpwdy1uss). The goal of cardiac rehabilitation is to monitor and improve the patient's cardiovascular status, thereby reversing the cardiac disease process and improving the patient's overall physical condition and quality of life. The success of cardiac rehabilitation is directly related to patient compliance. In addition to exercise, cardiac rehabilitation includes:

- managing stress
- controlling diet, nutrition, and weight
- reducing risk factors.

Advise your patient to use the U.S. Department of Agriculture's, ChooseMyPlate to make healthy food choices (https://www. choosemyplate.gov/)

Treatments for cardiomyopathy

You know
it's bad when I
need a VAD.

VAD

A ventricular assist device (VAD) is an implantable device that consists of a blood pump, cannulas, and a pneumatic or electrical drive console. The pump is synchronized to the patient's ECG and functions as the heart's ventricle. It decreases the heart's workload while increasing cardiac output.

Left VAD

A completely implanted left VAD is shown here.

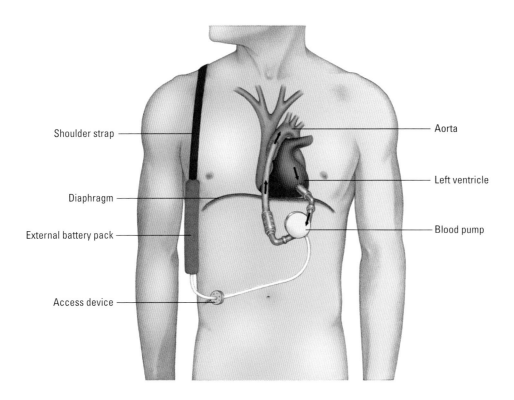

Shoulder strap

Diaphragm

External battery pack

Access device

Aorta

Left ventricle

Blood pump

Pump options

VADs are available as continuous flow or pulsatile pumps. A continuous flow pump fills continuously and returns blood to the aorta at a constant rate. A pulsatile pump may work in one of two ways:

1. It may fill during systole and pump blood into the aorta during diastole.
2. It may pump regardless of the patient's cardiac cycle.

Potential complications

Despite the use of anticoagulants, a VAD may cause thrombi formation, leading to pulmonary embolism or stroke. Other complications may include device malfunction (http://www.mayoclinic.org/tests-procedures/ventricular-assist-device/details/risks/cmc-20167078), heart failure, bleeding, cardiac tamponade, or infection.

A closer look at VADs

There are three types of VADs.

1

A right VAD provides pulmonary support by diverting blood from the failing right ventricle to the VAD, which then pumps the blood to the pulmonary circulation via the VAD connection to the left pulmonary artery.

2

With a left VAD, blood flows from the left ventricle to the VAD, which then pumps blood back to the body via the VAD connection to the aorta.

3

When a right and left VAD are used, it's referred to as a *biventricular VAD (BiVAD)*.

Thanks to my VAD, I'm all pumped up now.

Right VAD

Left VAD

Heart transplantation

In heart transplantation, a patient's failing heart is replaced with a donor heart. Used only to treat end-stage cardiac disease in patients who have poor quality of life and aren't expected to survive for more than 6 to 12 months, heart transplantation doesn't provide a cure.

Patients who receive donor hearts must be treated for rejection with monoclonal antibodies and potent immunosuppressants that can increase the risk of life-threatening infection.

 Photo op

Heart transplantation surgery

Before the donor's heart can be transplanted, the patient's failing heart is removed from his chest.

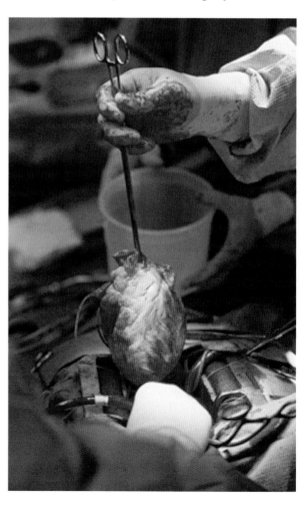

Heart to heart

The donor's heart

The donor's heart is removed after the surgeon cuts along these dissection lines.

Anterior view

The recipient's heart

Before it can be removed, the recipient's heart is resected along these lines.

The transplanted heart

The transplanted heart is sutured.

Valve treatments

Valve treatments are used to prevent heart failure in patients with valvular stenosis or insufficiency accompanied by severe, unmanageable symptoms. Depending on your patient's condition, he/she may undergo one of three types of valve surgery. When valve surgery isn't an option, percutaneous balloon valvuloplasty is used to enlarge the orifice of a stenotic heart valve, improving valvular function.

Valve replacement

In valve replacement, the natural heart valve is excised and a prosthetic valve is sutured in place.

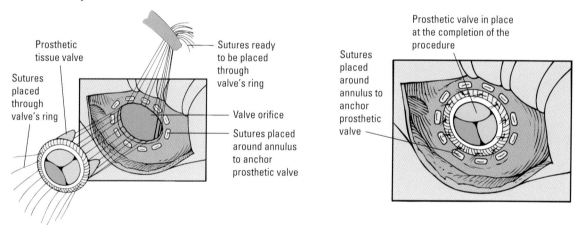

Prosthetic tissue valve

Sutures placed through valve's ring

Sutures ready to be placed through valve's ring

Valve orifice

Sutures placed around annulus to anchor prosthetic valve

Prosthetic valve in place at the completion of the procedure

Sutures placed around annulus to anchor prosthetic valve

Types of replacement valves

**Bileaflet valve
(St. Jude, mechanical)**

**Tilting-disk valve
(Medtronic-Hall, mechanical)**

**Porcine heterograft valve
(Carpentier-Edwards, tissue)**

Valve leaflet resection and repair

The section between the dashed
lines is excised.

The edges are approximated and sutured.

**The repair is finished off with
an annuloplasty ring.**

Commissurotomy

In commissurotomy, the thickened
leaflets are surgically separated. The
surgeon removes scar tissues and/or
calcium deposits from leaflets.

Percutaneous balloon valvuloplasty

During valvuloplasty, a surgeon inserts a small balloon catheter
through the skin at the femoral vein and advances it until it
reaches the affected valve. The balloon is then inflated, forcing
the valve opening to widen.

Commissurotomy of mitral valve

Catheter

Inflated balloon

Vascular repair

Vascular repair is a surgical option used to fix damaged or diseased vessels. Types of vascular repair include aortic aneurysm resection, bypass grafting, embolectomy, vena caval filter insertion, and endovascular stent grafting.

Aortic aneurysm resection

Aortic aneurysm resection involves removing an aneurysmal segment of the aorta. The surgeon first makes an incision to expose the aneurysm site. He/she then clamps the aorta, resects the aneurysm, and repairs the damaged portion of the aorta by sewing a prosthetic graft into place.

Bypass grafting

Bypass grafting serves to bypass an arterial obstruction resulting from arteriosclerosis. After exposing the affected artery, the surgeon anastomoses a synthetic or autogenous graft to divert blood flow around the occluded arterial segment. This illustration shows a femoropopliteal bypass.

Vena cava
Aorta
Aortic clamp
Kidney
Renal artery
Ureter
Incisions to open aneurysm sac
Common iliac artery
Iliac clamp

Occluded arterial segment
Graft

Aortic graft sewn into place

Embolectomy

To remove an embolism from an artery, a surgeon may perform an embolectomy by inserting a balloon-tipped indwelling catheter in the artery and passing it through the embolus (as shown below left). He/she then inflates the balloon and withdraws the catheter to remove the occlusion (as shown below right).

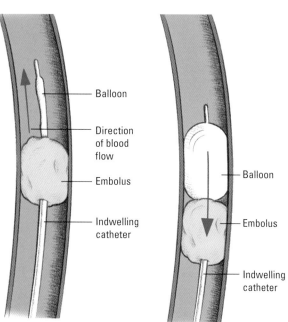

Vena caval filter insertion

A vena caval filter, or umbrella, traps emboli in the vena cava, preventing them from reaching the pulmonary vessels but allowing venous blood flow.

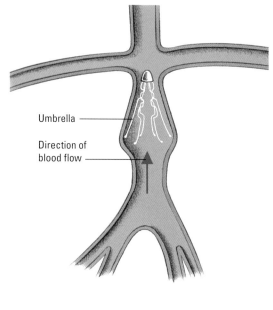

Endovascular stent grafting

Endovascular stent grafting is a minimally invasive procedure used to repair abdominal aortic aneurysm and other aneurysmal arteries by reinforcing the vessel walls. The surgeon uses fluoroscopic guidance to insert a delivery catheter with an attached compressed graft through a small incision into the femoral or iliac artery. The catheter is advanced into the aorta and positioned across the aneurysm below the renal arteries. The stent graft prevents blood from entering the aneurysmal area of the artery but maintains blood flow distally. This helps prevent the aneurysm from enlarging and possibly rupturing. The patient is instructed to walk within 24 hours and is discharged in 1 to 3 days after the procedure.

Aorto-iliac stent graft

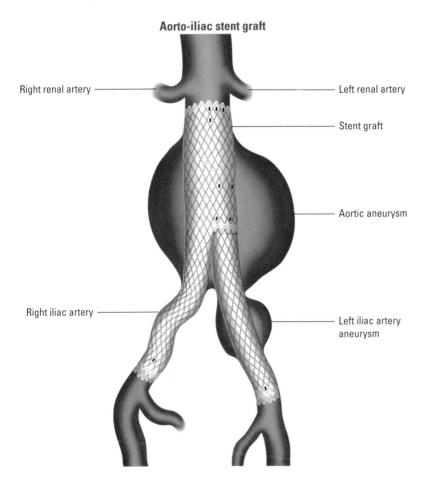

Right renal artery

Left renal artery

Stent graft

Aortic aneurysm

Right iliac artery

Left iliac artery aneurysm

Pericardiocentesis

Pericardiocentesis is an invasive procedure used to remove excess fluid that has accumulated in the pericardial sac (pericardial effusion). Rapid accumulation of pericardial fluid may require emergent pericardiocentesis in order to prevent circulatory collapse. Emergency equipment must be available.

A physician performs pericardiocentesis under fluoroscopic guidance in a cardiac catheterization laboratory or at the bedside with echocardiographic imaging. A pericardial aspiration needle with a three-way stopcock attached to a 50-ml syringe is used to aspirate the fluid from the pericardial sac. An alligator clip is attached to the aspirating needle, and an ECG machine is used to help check needle placement. At the end of the procedure, a catheter may be inserted and connected to a drainage bag for continuous drainage.

No wonder I'm depressed. My pericardium normally contains between 10 and 50 ml of fluid. Excess fluid puts pressure on me that depresses my function and leads to decreased cardiac output.

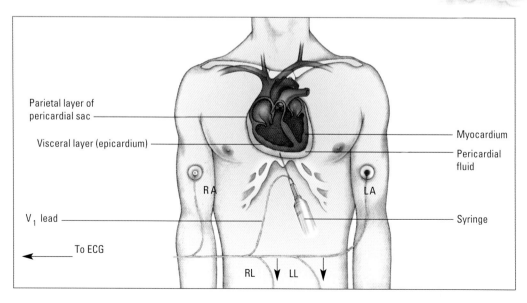

Parietal layer of pericardial sac

Visceral layer (epicardium)

Myocardium

Pericardial fluid

RA

LA

V_1 lead

Syringe

To ECG

RL   LL

Treatments for arrhythmias

Temporary pacing

Temporary pacing is used in arrhythmic emergencies, such as bradycardia and tachyarrhythmias, or other conduction system disturbances. Temporary pacemakers contain external, battery-powered pulse generators and a lead or electrode system.

Transcutaneous electrode placement

For a noninvasive temporary pacemaker, the two pacing electrodes are placed at heart level on the patient's chest and back, as shown. This type of pacemaker can be quickly applied in an emergency but is uncomfortable for the patient.

Monitoring electrode

Posterior pacing electrode

Anterior pacing electrode

Monitoring electrode

Pacer wires to pulse generator

Bradycardia algorithm

Bradycardia
Heart rate < 60 beats/min and inadequate for clinical condition

↓

- Maintain patent airway; assist breathing as needed.
- Give oxygen.
- Monitor ECG (identify rhythm), blood pressure, oximetry.
- Establish I.V. access.

↓

Signs or symptoms of poor perfusion caused by bradycardia (acute altered mental status, ongoing chest pain, hypotension, or other signs of shock)?

↓ ↓

| **ADEQUATE PERFUSION** | **POOR PERFUSION** |

↓ ↓

| Observe and monitor. | • Prepare for transcutaneous pacing; use without delay for high-degree block (type II second-degree block or third-degree AV block).
 • Consider atropine while awaiting pacer. May repeat to a total dose of 3 mg. If ineffective, begin pacing.
 • Consider epinephrine or dopamine infusion while awaiting pacer or if pacing is ineffective. |

↓

- Prepare for transvenous pacing.
- Treat contributing causes.
- Consider expert consultation.

Come equipped

Transvenous pulse generator

Sense meter registers every time the patient's heart beats.

Pace meter registers every pacing stimulus delivered to the heart.

Rate control sets the heart rate below which the pacemaker takes over.

Sensitivity control adjusts pacemaker sensitivity to the patient's heart rate. When the dial is set on ASYNC, the pacemaker delivers a set rate regardless of the patient's intrinsic rate.

Output control determines the number of milliamps of electricity sent to the heart.

On-off switch activates the pulse generator.

Battery compartment

Connector attaches the pacing wires to the pulse generator.

Temporary transvenous pacemaker

Transvenous pacing provides a more reliable pacing beat. This type of pacing is more comfortable for the patient because the pacing wire is inserted in the heart via a major vein.

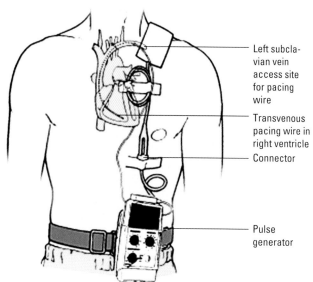

Left subclavian vein access site for pacing wire

Transvenous pacing wire in right ventricle

Connector

Pulse generator

Permanent pacing

A permanent pacemaker is a self-contained device that's surgically implanted in a pocket under the patient's skin. Pacemakers treat persistent bradyarrhythmias, complete heart block, congenital or degenerative heart diseases, Stokes-Adams syndrome, Wolff-Parkinson-White syndrome, and sick sinus syndrome. Pacing electrodes can be placed in the atria, the ventricles, or both chambers (atrioventricular sequential or dual chamber). Biventricular pacemakers also are available for cardiac resynchronization therapy in patients with heart failure.

Permanent pacemakers allow the patient's heart to beat on its own but keep the heartbeat from falling below a preset rate.

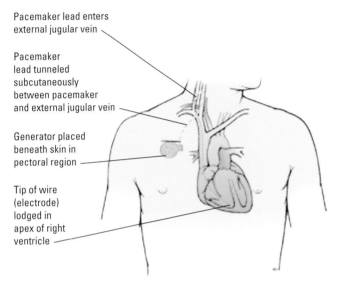

Pacemaker lead enters external jugular vein

Pacemaker lead tunneled subcutaneously between pacemaker and external jugular vein

Generator placed beneath skin in pectoral region

Tip of wire (electrode) lodged in apex of right ventricle

Biventricular pacemaker

A biventricular pacemaker utilizes three leads: one to pace the right atrium, one to pace the right ventricle, and one to pace the left ventricle. The left ventricular lead is placed in the coronary sinus. Both ventricles are paced at the same time, causing them to contract simultaneously, improving cardiac output.

Right atrial lead
Left ventricular lead

Right ventricular lead

Understanding pacemaker codes

First letter

Identifies heart chambers that are paced:
V = Ventricle
A = Atrium
D = Dual (ventricle and atrium)
O = None

> **memory board**
>
> The letters of the pacemaker code help you to understand what the pacemaker is doing. To remember this important ASPect of pacemaker coding, think of Cleopatra's ASP:
>
> **A**ssisted heart chamber
>
> **S**ensed heart chamber
>
> **P**acemaker response to intrinsic activity it sensed.

Second letter

Signifies the heart chamber where the pacemaker senses the intrinsic activity:
V = Ventricle
A = Atrium
D = Dual
O = None

> Asp-ed and answered. The most common pacing codes are VVI (single-chamber pacing) and DDD (dual-chamber pacing).

Third letter

Shows the pacemaker's response to the intrinsic electrical activity it senses in the atrium or ventricle:
T = Triggers pacing
I = Inhibits pacing
D = Dual (can be triggered or inhibited depending on the mode and where intrinsic activity occurs)
O = None (the pacemaker doesn't change its mode in response to sensed activity)

Pacemaker spikes

Pacemaker impulses — the stimuli that travel from the pacemaker to the heart — are visible on the patient's ECG tracing as spikes. Large or small pacemaker spikes appear above or below the isoelectric line. This example shows an atrial and a ventricular pacemaker spike.

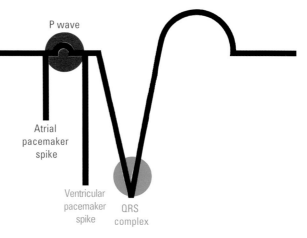

P wave

Atrial pacemaker spike

Ventricular pacemaker spike

QRS complex

Synchronized cardioversion

Synchronized cardioversion, also called *synchronized countershock*, is an elective or emergency procedure used to correct tachyarrhythmias. An electric current is delivered to the heart at a much lower energy level than used in defibrillation. The shock is synchronized to the peak R wave, causing immediate depolarization, interrupting reentry circuits, and allowing the SA node to resume control.

If the patient's cardiac rhythm changes to ventricular fibrillation during cardioversion, the modes can be switched from "synchronized" to "defibrillate" and the patient can be defibrillated immediately after the machine is recharged. The sync mode must be reset on the defibrillator after each synchronized cardioversion (most defibrillators automatically reset to an unsynchronized mode).

Choosing the correct cardioversion energy level

When choosing an energy level for cardioversion, try the lowest energy level first. If the arrhythmia isn't corrected, repeat the procedure using the next energy level until the arrhythmia is corrected or until you reach the highest energy level.

Monophasic energy doses for cardioversion

For unstable monomorphic ventricular tachycardia with a pulse	For unstable paroxysmal supraventricular tachycardia	For unstable atrial fibrillation with rapid ventricular response	For unstable atrial flutter with rapid ventricular response
100 joules	**50** joules	**100** joules	**50** joules
200 joules	**100** joules	**200** joules	**100** joules
300 joules	**200** joules	**300** joules	**200** joules
360 joules	**300** joules	**360** joules	**300** joules
	360 joules		**360** joules

The wise thing to do is use a stepwise approach to cardioversion.

Tachycardia algorithm

1

Tachycardia with pulses

2
- Assess and support ABCs as needed.
- Give oxygen.
- Monitor ECG (identify rhythm), blood pressure, oximetry.
- Identify and treat reversible causes.

4
Perform immediate synchronized cardioversion.
- Establish I.V. access and give sedation if patient is conscious; do not delay cardioversion.
- Consider expert consultation.
- If pulseless arrest develops, see pulseless arrest algorithm, page 256

Symptoms persist

3
Is patient stable?
Unstable signs include altered mental status, ongoing chest pain, hypotension, or other signs of shock.

Unstable

Stable

5
- Establish I.V. access.
- Obtain 12-lead ECG (when available) or rhythm strip.
Is QRS narrow?

Narrow (<0.12 sec)

6
Narrow QRS*
Is rhythm regular?

Wide (≥0.12 sec)

12
Wide QRS*
Is rhythm regular?
Expert consultation advised.

Regular

7
- Attempt vagal maneuvers.
- Give adenosine 6 mg rapid I.V. push. If no conversion, give 12 mg rapid I.V. push; may repeat 12-mg dose once.

Irregular

11
Irregular narrow-complex tachycardia
Probable atrial fibrillation or possible atrial flutter or multifocal atrial tachycardia
- Consider expert consultation.
- Control rate (diltiazem, beta-blockers; use beta-blockers with caution in pulmonary disease or heart failure).

Regular

13
If ventricular tachycardia or uncertain rhythm
- Amiodarone 150 mg I.V. over 10 min. Repeat as needed to maximum dosage of 2.2 g/24 hours.
- Prepare for elective synchronized cardioversion.

If SVT with aberrancy
- Give adenosine (go to box 7).

Irregular

14
If atrial fibrillation with aberrancy
- See Irregular narrow-complex tachycardia (box 11).

If preexcited atrial fibrillation (AF + WPW)
- Expert consultation advised.
- Avoid AV nodal blocking agents (adenosine, digoxin, diltiazem, verapamil).
- Consider antiarrhythmics (amiodarone 150 mg I.V. over 10 minutes).

If recurrent polymorphic VT
- Seek expert consultation.

If torsades de pointes
- Give magnesium (load with 1 to 2 g over 5 to 60 minutes, then infusion).

8
Does rhythm convert?
Note: Consider expert consultation.

Converts

9
If rhythm converts, probably reentry supraventricular tachycardia (SVT)
- Observe for recurrence.
- Treat recurrence with adenosine or longer-acting AV nodal blocking agents (such as diltiazem or beta-blockers).

Does not convert

10
If rhythm does NOT convert, possible atrial flutter, ectopic atrial tachycardia, or junctional tachycardia
- Control rate (diltiazem, beta-blockers; use beta-blockers with caution in pulmonary disease or heart failure).
- Treat underlying cause.
- Consider expert consultation.

*Note: If patient becomes unstable, go to box 4.

Implantable cardioverter-defibrillation

Implantable cardioverter-defibrillators (ICDs) are used for antiarrhythmic pacing, cardioversion, and defibrillation. Some defibrillators have the ability to pace the atrium and the ventricle, and some can perform biventricular pacing. A lead or leads are placed transvenously in the endocardium of the appropriate chambers. The lead connects to a generator box implanted in the right or left upper chest near the clavicle.

An ICD typically consists of a programmable pulse generator and an electrode. It detects ventricular bradyarrhythmias and tachyarrhythmias and responds with appropriate therapies.

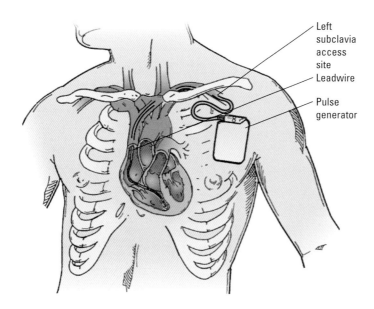

Left subclavia access site

Leadwire

Pulse generator

Types of ICD therapies

ICDs can deliver a range of therapies depending on the arrhythmia that's detected and how the device is programmed. These include antitachycardia pacing, cardioversion, defibrillation, and bradycardia pacing.

Therapy	What it does
Antitachycardia pacing	A series of small, rapid, electrical pacing pulses are used to interrupt ventricular tachycardia (VT) and return the heart to its normal rhythm.
Cardioversion	A low- or high-energy shock (up to 35 joules) is timed to the R wave to terminate VT and return the heart to its normal rhythm.
Defibrillation	A high-energy shock (up to 35 joules) to the heart is used to terminate ventricular fibrillation and return the heart to its normal rhythm.
Bradycardia pacing	Electrical pacing pulses are used when the heart's natural electrical signals are too slow. Most ICD systems can pace one chamber (VVI pacing) of the heart at a preset rate. Some systems will sense and pace both chambers (DDD pacing).

Radiofrequency ablation

Radiofrequency ablation is used to treat arrhythmias in patients who don't respond to antiarrhythmic drugs or cardioversion. During the procedure, a special catheter is inserted in a vein and advanced to the heart. After the source of the arrhythmia is identified, radiofrequency energy destroys the abnormal electrical impulses or conduction pathway. The tissue that's destroyed can no longer conduct electrical impulses.

Types of ablation

AV node ablation

If a rapid arrhythmia originates above the AV node, the AV node may be destroyed to block impulses from reaching the ventricles. A pacemaker may then be required to stimulate the ventricles.

The radiofrequency ablation catheter is directed to the AV node.

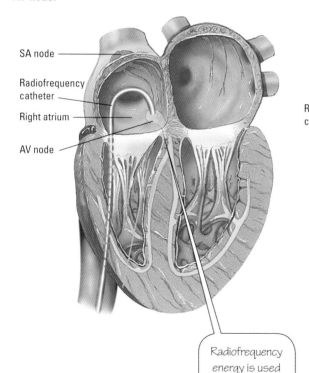

SA node

Radiofrequency catheter

Right atrium

AV node

Radiofrequency energy is used to destroy the AV node.

Pulmonary vein ablation

If a pulmonary vein is the source of the arrhythmia, such as in atrial fibrillation, radiofrequency energy is used to destroy the tissue in the area of the atrium that connects to the pulmonary vein. The scar that forms blocks impulses from firing within the pulmonary vein, preventing the arrhythmia.

The radiofrequency catheter is directed to the base of the pulmonary vein.

Pulmonary vein

SA node

Radiofrequency catheter

Radiofrequency energy is used to destroy the tissue where the atrium connects to the pulmonary vein.

Pulseless arrest algorithm

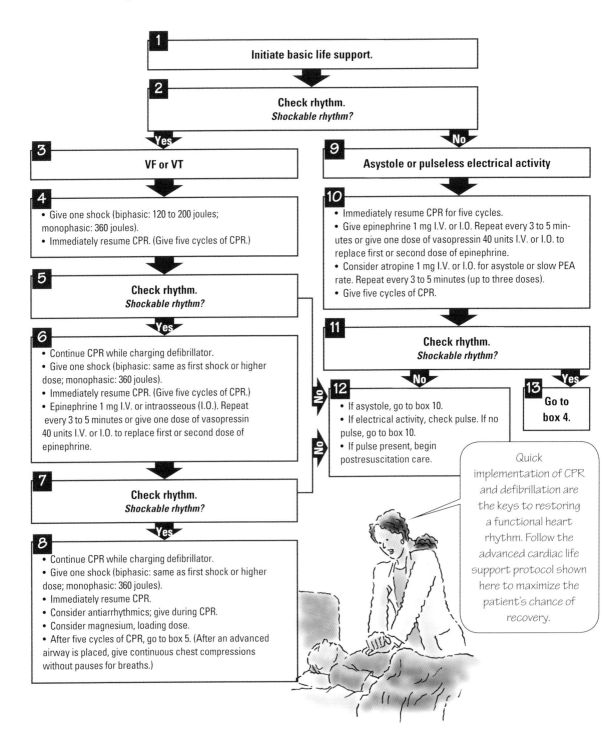

1 Initiate basic life support.

2 Check rhythm.
Shockable rhythm?

— Yes →

3 VF or VT

4
- Give one shock (biphasic: 120 to 200 joules; monophasic: 360 joules).
- Immediately resume CPR. (Give five cycles of CPR.)

5 Check rhythm.
Shockable rhythm?

— Yes →

6
- Continue CPR while charging defibrillator.
- Give one shock (biphasic: same as first shock or higher dose; monophasic: 360 joules).
- Immediately resume CPR. (Give five cycles of CPR.)
- Epinephrine 1 mg I.V. or intraosseous (I.O.). Repeat every 3 to 5 minutes or give one dose of vasopressin 40 units I.V. or I.O. to replace first or second dose of epinephrine.

7 Check rhythm.
Shockable rhythm?

— Yes →

8
- Continue CPR while charging defibrillator.
- Give one shock (biphasic: same as first shock or higher dose; monophasic: 360 joules).
- Immediately resume CPR.
- Consider antiarrhythmics; give during CPR.
- Consider magnesium, loading dose.
- After five cycles of CPR, go to box 5. (After an advanced airway is placed, give continuous chest compressions without pauses for breaths.)

9 Asystole or pulseless electrical activity

— No →

10
- Immediately resume CPR for five cycles.
- Give epinephrine 1 mg I.V. or I.O. Repeat every 3 to 5 minutes or give one dose of vasopressin 40 units I.V. or I.O. to replace first or second dose of epinephrine.
- Consider atropine 1 mg I.V. or I.O. for asystole or slow PEA rate. Repeat every 3 to 5 minutes (up to three doses).
- Give five cycles of CPR.

11 Check rhythm.
Shockable rhythm?

No →

12
- If asystole, go to box 10.
- If electrical activity, check pulse. If no pulse, go to box 10.
- If pulse present, begin postresuscitation care.

Yes →

13 Go to box 4.

No / No

Quick implementation of CPR and defibrillation are the keys to restoring a functional heart rhythm. Follow the advanced cardiac life support protocol shown here to maximize the patient's chance of recovery.

Cardiopulmonary resuscitation

Effective CPR requires compressions that are hard, fast, accurately placed, and allow complete chest recoil. If a second rescuer arrives, chest compressions should be continuous and ventilation should be provided at 8 to 10 breaths/ minute during compressions.

Photo op

Performing one-person CPR

1 After initiating the emergency response team or calling for a defibrillator when a patient is unresponsive, position the patient supine on a hard surface and open the airway. Then, check for adequate breathing for 10 seconds.

2 Perform ventilation with two breaths that make the chest rise, at 1 second per breath. If ineffective, reposition the airway and retry.

3 Palpate the carotid pulse for no more than 10 seconds. Unless a definite pulse is felt, initiate chest compressions.

4 Place hands one on top of the other on the lower half of the sternum between the nipples, with elbows locked. Compress the chest 2′ (or one-third the depth of the chest) at a rate of 100 to 120 compressions per minute, keeping your hands on the chest. Allow equal time for compression and full chest recoil. Continue for 30 compressions, then give 2 ventilations and resume compressions quickly for five cycles (2 minutes) before rechecking the pulse (http://eccguidelines.heart.org/wp-content/uploads/2015/10/2015-AHA-Guidelines-Highlights-English.pdf)

Defibrillation

In defibrillation, electrode paddles direct an electric current through the patient's heart, causing the myocardium to depolarize, which in turn encourages the SA node to resume control of the heart's electrical activity. Because some arrhythmias can cause death, the success of defibrillation depends on early recognition and intervention.

Placing the paddles

During defibrillation, place the paddles as shown. During cardiac surgery, smaller paddles may be placed directly on the myocardium.

Come equipped

The defibrillator

How to perform defibrillation

To perform external defibrillation on an adult, give one shock. The number of joules to give depends on the machine being used:
• monophasic — 360 joules
• biphasic — see manufacturer's instructions
• automated external defibrillator — preset by the machine.

If your patient doesn't have a pulse after defibrillation, quickly resume CPR for 2 minutes and then reattempt defibrillation.

ECG monitor

Paddles

SYNC/ASYNC button

Pacer output

Mode selection

Pacer sensitivity

Shock discharge

Automated external defibrillation

An automated external defibrillator (AED) has a cardiac rhythm analysis system that interprets the patient's cardiac rhythm and gives the operator step-by-step directions on how to proceed. This device was designed to allow laypeople with CPR and AED training to initiate care in an emergency until medical staff arrive.

Come equipped

The AED

An AED has a "quick-look" feature that analyzes a patient's heart rhythm. This feature allows you to visualize the heart's rhythm by pushing a button after the electrodes are connected. Then, the defibrillator audibly and visually prompts you to deliver a shock, if needed.

Quick-look screen

Shock button

Electrodes

Face shield

Matchmaker

Match the equipment in the pictures at right with the procedures for which they're used.

1. _____

2. _____

A. Temporary pacing

B. Automated external defibrillation

C. Valve replacement

3. _____

Photo finish

Number these photos in the correct step-by-step order for performing CPR.

Suggested references

Montalescot, G., Sechtem, U., Achenbach, S., Andreotti, F., Arden, C.,, ... Zamorano, J.L. 2013 ESC Guidelines on the Management of Stable Coronary Artery Disease: The Task Force on the Management of Stable Coronary Artery Disease of the European Society of Cardiology. *European Heart Journal* 34: 2949–3003, 2013.

https://www.drugs.com/drug-class/aldosterone-receptor-antagonists.html

http://www.mayoclinic.org/diseases-conditions/high-blood-pressure/in-depth/diuretics/art-20048129

https://www.uptodate.com/contents/treatment-of-resistant-hypertension

http://www.healthline.com/health/anticoagulant-and-antiplatelet-drugs#overview16

http://www.heart.org/HEARTORG/Conditions/More/CardiacRehab/What-is-Cardiac-Rehabilitation_UCM_307049_Article.jsp#.WQkpwdy1uss

https://www.choosemyplate.gov/

http://www.mayoclinic.org/tests-procedures/ventricular-assist-device/details/risks/cmc-20167078

http://eccguidelines.heart.org/wp-content/uploads/2015/10/2015-AHA-Guidelines-Highlights-English.pdf

Index